FIT TO SERVE

STEPHANIE DEAN

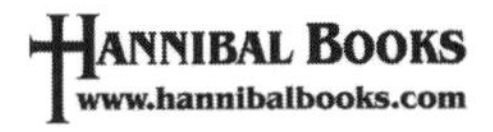

Published by
Hannibal Books
PO Box 461592
Garland, TX 75046-1592
Copyright Stephanie Dean 2008
All Rights Reserved
Printed in the United States of America
by Lightning Source, LaVergne, TN
Cover design by Dennis Davidson
Illustrations by Greg Crull
Except where otherwise indicated, all Scripture taken from the
Holy Bible, *New International Version*, copyright 1973, 1978, 1984
by International Bible Society.

ISBN 978-1-934749-29-6
Library of Congress Control Number: 2008934894

TO ORDER ADDITIONAL COPIES FOR $14.95 EACH (ADD $4.00 SHIPPING FOR FIRST BOOK,
$1.00 FOR EACH ADDITIONAL BOOK) CONTACT
Hannibal Books
PO BOX 461592
GARLAND, TX 75046-1592
www.hannibalbooks.com
800-747-0738 (toll free)

Dedicated

to my parents,

Bob and Ellen Dean

in appreciation for their surrender to and service of our Lord.
I love you.

Acknowledgements

To Julie, Carol, and Don

Without your work, we would not have this Bible study.
Thank you for your willingness to serve on a team together. Your expertise, your love for the Lord, and your desire to build up the church gave me strength (Eccl. 4:12). The church works best together.

To the local church

Thanks for valuing discipleship and for letting me see that God links the secular with the sacred. Thanks to Lake Pointe Church, Rockwall, TX. You let us serve. Thanks to Northlake Baptist Church, Garland, TX. You invested through the years.

To Hannibal Books

Thanks to Louis and Kay Moore and Katie Welch for allowing this book to be in print.
Kay, thanks for using your much-appreciated editing skills and for your patience.

Contents

Note

This book was written as a reference manual only. It is not a medical manual, nor is it a substitute for medical treatment from your physician or health professional. Please seek immediate and competent medical help if you suspect that you have a medical problem. Nutrition and exercise needs change depending on each individual's age, gender, diet, physical-fitness level, and medical history. This information was written to aid you in making informed decisions about your health.

The authors, publishers, and distributors are not liable for any health impairment, injury, or accident befalling any reader of this book or any health impairment injury, or accident that may befall any person using techniques or guidelines from this book.

Letter to Readers

Dear Group Member,

Welcome to *Fit to Serve*. I am so glad you joined us for this six-week Bible study on spiritual disciplines and wellness. This Bible study uniquely links the spiritual and physical health of a Christ-follower. It keeps our spiritual health prominent while we continue to value physical health.

This book represents the joint effort of four authors—all believers in Christ: fitness experts Don and Carol Mathus, nutritionist Julie Bender, and myself, a dietitian. Our goal—to build up the church so it can fulfill its purpose in the world. To accomplish this, we focus on the individual—you. We hope the church—the Body of Christ—will function at optimum capacity, which means all of us strive to be spiritually and physically fit to serve. Therefore, for six weeks we combine spiritual disciplines, nutrition, and exercise. This study will get you moving and keep you on the road. When you read the first-person references in the Bible study, they relate to my life experiences. Don, Carol, and Julie have taken turns writing the "health bites"—the nutrition and wellness sections that follow the Bible studies. They also took turns writing the health and fitness emphasis in the weekly lessons that you will hear your leader present during your group sessions.

For the next six weeks, for five days each, you will be asked to read the study materials, complete the questions asked, and then attend a group meeting at which you will share about what God taught you during your weekly study. I encourage you to complete your daily work so the study will have the most meaning for you.

Gear up for the journey—you just stepped out on a road to a healthier you. We are on a journey home—a journey we began when we believed Jesus was who He claimed to be—the Son of God, fully God and fully man, humanity's only way of salvation (John 14:6). This is a journey that keeps us focused on getting home. Our home we recognize is in heaven; there our loyalty lies, too (Phil. 3:12-21). We don't know what roadblocks you may encounter during these six weeks. We pray, however, that God will sustain you along the way. We hope all of us persevere in our faith and live as good stewards of our health.

Put on your walking shoes. We will take this study at a nice clip. Are you ready? Let the journey begin.

For the health of the Body,

Stephanie Dean

What others are saying about this book:

Fit to Serve provides insight into two important areas of one's life: physical health and spiritual health. The authors propose logical, fact-based solutions to weight-control issues as well as insightful guidance for spiritual growth. This book offers reliable, practical, and timely information about staying healthy in a busy world.

LuAnn Soliah, Ph.D., R.D.

Fit to Serve is more than a Bible study; it's a complete workout, spiritually and physically. Linking spiritual disciplines with nutritional and physical wellness is highly creative—it leads to an all-around fitness.

Ty Daughtry, Pastor to Adults
Lake Pointe Church, Rockwall, TX

Weekly Bible Studies

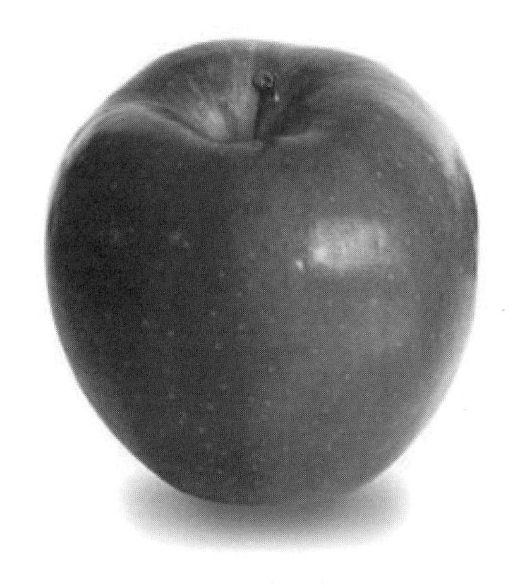

9/6/15

Week 1 - Day 1

Secular or Sacred?

Memory Verse:

All Scripture is God-breathed and is useful for teaching, rebuking, correcting and training in righteousness (2 Tim. 3:16 NIV).

"Mr. Wilberforce, we understand you are having problems choosing to do the work of God or the work of a political activist.

"We humbly suggest you can do both."

The lines are from *Amazing Grace*, the movie recounting the story of William Wilberforce as he spearheaded the abolitionist movement in England. In a pivotal scene, John Newton, author of the hymn, *Amazing Grace*, and Wilberforce's pastor, encouraged William to combine the two. "Wilber, you have work to do."

Wilberforce struggled to choose between the secular and the sacred.

What about you? Have you ever faced a similar challenge?

A perceived dichotomy

Early on I felt led to pursue a career in healthcare. I believed God directed this decision. However, at the end of college things changed. I sensed a calling toward either vocational or bivocational ministry. Yet several factors caused me to hesitate to accept. One was a blossoming career in nutrition. After I graduated, I accepted an internship in Dallas and headed off without making a commitment about ministry.

My year as a dietetic intern stood as a high point—a completely wonderful experience. However, during this time God continued to confirm ministry. I knew this would impact the rest of my decisions.

After I declared a call to ministry and a new direction which included seminary training, I faced a challenge. What about nutrition? Had God led me down the healthcare path just to teach me a few lessons or for another purpose? On seeking advice from friends and family, I received a variety of responses. They typically fell into three categories:

1. Quit nutrition and pursue ministry full-time.
2. Work as a dietitian to pay my way through seminary and possibly ministry.
3. Work as a dietitian and plan to use nutrition as a platform for ministry.

From the start I liked the third option best. *Yet how do I accomplish this?* I wondered.

A Christian worldview

Once I began pursuing ministry, God did open up more opportunities to serve Him. Most of the time people requested that I link the two. This required me to investigate the connection between our physical and spiritual health.

In the end this investigation brought me back to a complex yet foundational concept: an individual who follows Christ seeks to filter all aspects of life through Christian faith. Our faith works in unity with our life's work. We do not build walls to separate the secular and sacred in our lives. Instead we seek the glorification of God through even the mundane aspects of life. The practice of spiritual disciplines plays a key role in developing a Christian worldview.

First we must know God's truth. For this reason we begin our first week with the spiritual discipline of studying Scripture.

Breathed by God

What would you say if someone were to ask you, *why* or *how do you practice the spiritual discipline of studying God's Word?*

As I learn more about this discipline, I find many sources frequently cite 2 Timothy 3:16. The two reasons this verse remains a favorite lie in its ability to explain why we can look to Scripture and *how* it actually helps the Christ-follower live according to God's will.

Because this verse is so useful, studying and memorizing it will help us. This is what I pray we will accomplish this week.

Each day we will study one part of the verse. Today we will focus on *All Scripture is God-breathed.* This short phrase brims with information to help us understand why we can look to Scripture as the Word of God. First, let us look at the expression *God-breathed—theopneustos* in the Greek language. Paul coins this word; the only time we find it in the Bible is here in 2 Timothy 3:16. This compound word combines two terms. The first term, *theos,* means *God* and usually refers to the one true God. The second part, *pneu,* means "to blow (of wind)"[1]. The English language does not have a word that equally translates *theopneustos*. Therefore, depending on your Bible's translation, you may find this Greek word recorded as *God-breathed, inspired by God*, or *breathed out by God.*

Theopneustos carries with it the role of God in the creation of the words.[2] We know the Holy Spirit used the prophets or those in the apostles' circle to write Scripture (2 Pet. 1:19-21). Yet the meaning of this term in 2 Timothy 3:16 confirms that even though individuals wrote down the text, we can take it as a word from God.

Because God inspired Scripture, it carries greater authority than other books do. For though human beings penned it, it exists as the inspired words of God. Authority springs from its source—God.

How does the inspiration of the Bible affect your personal study and application of Scripture?

____

____

Savoring Scripture

Imagine your favorite food. Think of the smell. Visualize it. Remember the flavor. Have I piqued your appetite? If one evening you experience an intense craving for this food, what would you do? Often people say nothing satisfies them until they have eaten a particular food they crave. When you think of Scripture, does the very mention of it create a similar longing? Would you respond to the urge the same way?

The psalmist tells us that God's Word is more pleasurable than food is. *They are more precious than gold, than much pure gold; they are sweeter than honey, than honey from the comb* (Ps. 19:10). *How sweet are your words to my taste, sweeter than honey to my mouth!* (Ps. 119:103). Scripture brings us both nourishment and enjoyment spiritually.

Below write down one of your favorite Bible verses. If you don't have a favorite yet, then simply write down a prayer that the Holy Spirit soon will bring His Word to life for you.

____

____

____

Take a moment and think about the authority of God's Word, for your view of authority often correlates with how you apply Scripture to your life. Then answer the questions on the next page.

On average, how many days a week do you read the Bible?
1 2 3 4 5 6 7

How many minutes do you spend reading God's Word?
_____________ minutes

Do you memorize Scripture? If so, please write down the last verse you memorized.
____
____
____

Rank your response to the questions below.
(1= highly unlikely, 2= unlikely, 3=neutral, 4=likely, 5=very likely)

__________ When I am stressed about relationships, I read God's Word.
__________ When I am overwhelmed at work, I read the Bible.
__________ When I struggle with sin, I read God's Word.
__________ When life goes great, I read Scripture.
__________ Before I make a big decision, I read God's Word.
__________ To help fight temptation, I read or memorize Scripture.
__________ At church I regularly look up verses to check the validity of the teaching/preaching.
__________ To encourage a friend, I point the person to Scripture.

Eating your favorite food far exceeds hearing someone else tell you how great it tastes. In the same way, studying God's Word for yourself brings delight and sweetness with the practice of it.

As we look at studying the Bible, I encourage you to schedule a time to study God's Word. For just as food provides nourishment for life, studying the Bible feeds us spiritually as we follow Christ.

Write down the place and time you plan to study Scripture.
@ Home 10pm - 10:30pm
____

Read either Psalm 19 or 119. Write down what benefits the psalmist lists as gain from studying and applying Scripture.
____
____
____
____

9/7/15

Day 1 Health Bite

God designed each one of us for wellness. He desires us to care for the bodies and souls He has graciously given us, so that we may live each day to its fullest. Our responsibility is to be mindful of the gift of food He has created for our enjoyment. In our current culture this is not always easy. The vision of this nutrition and wellness section is to equip and encourage you to achieve a healthier lifestyle and relationship with the one thing we physically cannot live without—food.

Just as reading your Bible takes discipline, as you seek to learn more about your heavenly Father and His design for your life, discipline is necessary to care for the body He has entrusted to you. That does not mean we have to succumb to our culture and aspire to look like the unrealistic images we see on the pages of our favorite magazines. God created us in all different shapes and sizes; that is what makes us unique. As you take your first step toward better health and wellness, take some time to reflect on the following questions.

On a scale of 1 to 10, how do you view your current "health"?
(1=very unhealthy 10= extremely healthy) ________________________________

In the above question, why did you give yourself the rating you did?

____

____

In what ways would you like to see your health improve throughout the next year?
(Ex: lose weight, control diabetes or high blood pressure, prevent disease, gain more energy or sleep, reduce stress)

____

____

____

What is motivating you to consider making changes that will positively affect your health?

____

____

____

Week 1 - Day 2

Teaching, Truth, and Thelma

Memory Verse:

All Scripture is God-breathed and is useful for teaching, rebuking, correcting and training in righteousness (2 Tim. 3:16 NIV).

During Super Summer Youth Camp before my sophomore year in high school, God's Word grabbed my attention. One day during the morning devotionals I struggled to study Scripture. My thoughts kept drifting to a current crisis. Since I was 4, I had scoliosis and received appropriate medical treatment, yet the physicians told me of a recent development—I needed surgery that year. Pain was not the issue; it was the scar. For an adolescent girl in an image-driven culture, a scar is a huge factor.

I flipped haphazardly through the psalms; the word *radiant* caught my eye. This word linked the scar and the Scripture. God seemed to whisper, "Stephanie, do you want to be *radiant*, or will you settle for *beautiful*?" God knew the real issue lay deeper than pain, scars, and appearance. He met me where I was.

Then I read the rest of Psalm 34; God spoke to my heart about fear. God doesn't always remove us from the circumstance but from the fears that disable us. He replaces it with a fear and an awe of Him. I immediately decided to make Psalm 34 my life motto.

On Sunday night after camp, Thelma, one of the senior adults at church, sat down next to me and asked what God taught me. I told her about Psalm 34. She listened quietly. When I finished telling her the story, she said, "You know, that is interesting, because Psalm 34 is a special chapter to me, too. You may not know this. The day before you were born, my daughter died suddenly; God comforted me with Psalm 34. When you were born, the doctors told your parents they did not expect you to survive; the church sent around a prayer chain. I prayed Psalm 34. Each time you have been in the hospital or sick, this was my prayer." Then Thelma opened her Bible and pointed to my name written by several verses in Psalm 34. These notations included the dates she prayed for me.

In that moment, God's Word became real in a way I had never experienced. Not only did I serve a God who was holy and powerful in the past, but He transcends all time. He showed Himself as an almighty, sovereign God to King David, Thelma, and me. Wow! Don't we serve an amazing God? A year ago my dad preached Thelma's funeral.

He used her Bible and told of how she, a woman of prayer, encouraged other believers with God's Word.

The Holy Spirit uses Scripture to teach His children truth. This still remains one of my favorite stories of how God brought truth to real life in the midst a crisis. Let's look at this psalm a little closer to see the context of David's crisis and enduring truth about God.

Have you had a time in your life in which God used Scripture and/or another believer who studies God's Word with you to teach you an important lesson? If so, describe below.

____

____

____

____

David on the run

Turn to and read Psalm 34. Look at a note included before the first verse. Here the Bible tells us the circumstance in which David writes. Turn to and read 1 Samuel 21:10-15.

At this time Samuel has already anointed David as king. But Saul remains in control of the throne. David serves Saul faithfully. Yet because of Saul's jealousy, he seeks to kill David (1 Sam. 18). Therefore David's only hope of survival means running for his life. In fact, the threat becomes so great that David goes into enemy land—specifically to Philistine territory. Not long after he arrives, the Philistines recognize his identity. They remember this mighty warrior and decide to hold him hostage (1 Sam. 21:13)[1]. David cunningly decides to act insane. Thus King Achish, also known as Abimelech, allows him to leave.

Act insane

During college I took a self-defense class. Within the first week the one male student dropped the course; it ended up as a time in which a group of non-threatening young women practiced escape moves, kicks, and punches. Each time we left the class, our adrenaline ran high; our eyes scanned the environment for suspicious individuals.

Near the end of the semester our professor sat us down for a talk. In a serious tone he stated that if we were attacked, the perpetrator would most likely have the advantage over us in strength. He said, "Ladies, you have a few means you can use to fight back.

First you have speed. Try to avoid a confrontation when possible. Second, if you must fight, strike with accuracy. Third, many of you possess the element of surprise; hopefully, the perpetrator will not expect you to fight back." Then he added, "If these three don't work, act insane. They may think you are crazier than they are and leave you alone."

We found this quite amusing. Of course we hope we never have to apply what we learned. But I noticed a correlation between what he taught us and David's plan in Philistine territory. Who knows? Maybe our professor got the idea from 1 Samuel.

Developing doctrine

David's plan and my professor's advice may both work in a crisis. But when David writes Psalm 34, he does not give us details about how or when one is to act insane. Instead, the Holy Spirit inspires David to write about a better way to deal with a crisis. This psalm contains a lesson about God, fear, and living a righteous life. Scripture offers us a better teaching.

All 66 books of the Bible can provide instruction. They help us to develop personal doctrines, mission statements, and worldviews.

Studying Scripture involves digging deeper into the text. Vehicles such as researching the context aid in our identification of the main themes in a Bible passage. Without taking the time to study and work, we may develop unfounded doctrines, mission statements, and worldviews. The benefits of studying the Bible far outweigh the time and effort of this discipline.

Today, since we already discussed the context, outline the main sections in Psalm 34 and identify the main themes or truths. Then write a summary statement of how this applies to your life.

____

____

____

____

____

The best thing to do is prayerfully seek God as you study the Bible. As Christ-followers, we have the Holy Spirit to guide us (1 Cor. 2:6-16). Spend time thinking about a verse or section. This involves looking at a passage both in detail (verse by verse) and with the big picture in mind (main concepts of entire passage).

Day 2 Health Bite

To enjoy health and vigor later in life, people ideally will cultivate wellness while they are young. For just a minute let us tell you a little about ourselves, how we became interested in fitness, and why we are so passionate about it.

Carol's story:
I grew up playing outdoors, riding my bike, swimming, and snow-skiing. My enthusiasm for being physically active led me to a career as a physical-education teacher. I discovered running as a way to maintain my weight, reduce stress, and as a time to think and pray. I also enjoy riding my bike and lifting weights.

Don's story:
After an active youth and a stint in the army, physical education seemed to be the obvious field of study for me in college. Part-time YMCA work and coaching youth sports teams confirmed my choice. The course work and lab time emphasized how crucial our personal fitness is to the quality of our life. Fitness became a way of life for me. Through almost 40 years of teaching, I still enjoy my running, bike riding, and weight training.

Your story:
Think about your own health status at this time. Do you have limitations and/or health issues that you need to address? If so, a physician's clearance for exercise is recommended. Take a few minutes and fill out the Personal Health Inventory on the next page. And remember, *Whether you eat or drink, or whatever you do, do everything for the glory of God* (1 Cor. 10:31).

Challenge:: Walk for 5 minutes
Do 2 push-ups
Do 10 abdominal crunches

Personal Health Inventory

1. Describe your health:

2. What are you currently doing to promote your own fitness?

3. Would you consider yourself underweight, overweight, or within normal range?

4. With what personal health and fitness habits are you happy?

5. In the next six weeks what health and fitness changes would you like to achieve?

6. What long-term goals (between six weeks and one year) would you like to achieve?

Week 1 - Day 3

A Loving Rebuke

Memory Verse:

All Scripture is God-breathed and is useful for teaching, rebuking, correcting and training in righteousness (2 Tim. 3:16 NIV).

Today we study how Scripture can bring rebuke or reproof to our lives. The Greek word used in this verse is *elenchos,* which means "certainty, proof; rebuke, reproof."[1]

Describe what you think when you hear the word *rebuke.*

____

____

Our memory verse for this week lists reproof as a benefit of God's Word. A biblical rebuke occurs out of love and contains a desire for restoration. Without rebuke, we will likely continue in our sin. This will lead to our destruction.

A Word from God

In the Old Testament, God regularly uses a prophet to send a word to His people. We find the Old Testament filled with stories of prophets such as Samuel, Nathan, Hosea, Jonah, and more. Today, as we study *rebuke,* we will focus on the prophet Nathan and King David.

Turn to and read 2 Samuel 11:1-27. We find ourselves with the infamous story of David and Bathsheba. Take a moment and list all of the sins David commits.

____

____

____

In 2 Samuel 11:1 we find David taking a break from fulfilling his typical duties. *In the spring, at the time when kings go off to war, David sent Joab out with the king's men and the whole Israelite army. They destroyed the Ammonites and besieged Rabbah. <u>But David remained in Jerusalem</u>.* [Emphasis mine] (2 Sam. 11:1).

David's choice to stay back in Jerusalem raises a red flag. Warning—danger lies ahead!

When David chooses to stay home, he takes the first step off the path of following God's will. He lets up on his God-given duty as king. He chooses laziness. For a moment let's look back at the book of Proverbs. King Solomon, the son of David and Bathsheba, writes most of this book.

Proverbs 18:9 states that laziness destroys or wastes.[2] *One who is slack in his work is brother to one who destroys* (Prov. 18:9). A choice to "be slack" may seem harmless. But in 2 Samuel we find that David's choice to stay in Jerusalem increases his vulnerability to temptation and sin.

Read 2 Samuel 12:1-25. Verse 1 tells us that the Lord sends Nathan to give David a parable and a rebuke. The first three words, *The Lord sent*, hold importance. This message is from God and not from people.

The Lord has provided a Word for us today; occasionally we are called to confront a brother or sister who lives contrary to Scripture (1 Cor. 5). But our only appeal for them to change must rest in God's Word. We must seek a fully restored relationship. The message must come from the Lord and not from people.

The Lord sends Nathan to tell a *story*. Why do you think He does this?

____

____

____

In 2 Samuel 12:5-6, David condemns himself when he pronounces judgment on the rich man. Have you ever read a Scripture passage and thought what a pertinent message this would be for a friend or family member? From David's example we see that when identifying a need for biblical reproof, we first must examine ourselves (Luke 6:37-42).

Nathan then gives David a direct rebuke from the Lord (2 Sam. 12:7-10). The Lord lists David's consequences for his sin (2 Sam. 12:11-12).

How does David respond to the Lord's message of reproof and pronouncement of punishment?

____

David does evil and displeases the Lord. When he is confronted, he finally stops trying to hide his sin. David acknowledges his personal action and the impact of his sin against the Lord. He accepts the consequences. David's fall is a big one. But God provides restoration when David receives the rebuke and repents.

As you read the story of Nathan and David, what lessons do you learn about reproof? Describe.

____

____

____

____

David writes Psalm 51 about the time he is involved in the events of 2 Samuel 11-12. Take a moment and outline this psalm. It can serve as a guide for repentance when God rebukes us through His Word.

Many refer to King David as *a man after God's own heart*. This characteristic influences God's choice of him as king (1 Sam. 16:7). Even during valleys in David's life he wants faithfully to seek the Lord with a pure heart (Ps. 51:10-12). God accepts David's genuine confession and repentance and grants him forgiveness (2 Sam. 12:13b). In the New Testament the Apostle Paul describes David as a man after God's heart because of David's obedience (Acts 13:22). When God rebukes us, will we respond the same way as David did?

Day 3 Health Bite

Long-term weight loss is a goal for millions of men and women, but it is very challenging because it involves changing our daily habits! Altering habits involves effort and discipline. It requires a shift in how we organize priorities. In our culture, lack of "willpower" often is associated with overeating and weight gain. However, failure to obtain a healthy weight may be associated with lack of accurate nutrition education and counseling or may be complicated by emotional eating issues or lack of resources needed to help initiate healthy habits.

Before we set out to modify any behavior, identifying potential challenges that may affect success is important! A hectic schedule that does not allow for timely meals, tempting sweets in the office break room, the habit of polishing off leftovers, or the intense craving for sweets are very common challenges. "Willpower" is not the only thing that will tackle these behaviors. Instead, to allow change to occur you can identify and implement strategies that will overcome these daily events!

I urge you to identify the obstacles that may affect your decision to select the type of food that would provide optimal energy and nourishment. To overcome these challenges, place health and wellness on your "priority list"! Keep in mind—taking time for personal self-care can lead to increased energy, confidence, and stamina to be a better spouse, parent, co-worker, and ultimately a faithful follower of Christ!

What are some "barriers" or "obstacles" to forming healthy eating habits?

____

____

____

List at least one possible solution around each barrier.

____

____

____

Identify one change you are thinking about making to improve your health.

____

____

How can you use Scripture to help encourage you? (Matt. 7:7)

____

____

Week 1 - Day 4

The Tale of Spring City

Memory Verse:

All Scripture is God-breathed and is useful for teaching, rebuking, correcting and training in righteousness (2 Tim. 3:16 NIV).

Far, far away, the owner of a large plot of land gave rights to 1,000 acres and a natural spring to charter a town called Spring City. His only guideline required that the city maintain an arboretum as a beautiful reminder of his love for creation and the people of their town. This arboretum became its primary economic resource.

A drought fell over the town of Spring City; yet, since it had rights to a deep natural spring, it continued to provide water for the people and the arboretum. At the beginning of the drought the city council interviewed and hired a caretaker. The city designated him as manager of the natural spring and its maintenance and safekeeping.

A maiden in Spring City owned a yearly pass to the arboretum. She soon befriended the caretaker; they regularly met at the spring to talk. One summer afternoon the caretaker and maiden decided to go swimming in the spring. They splashed around and shrilled with excitement over their exhilarating swim. From then on, they met to go swimming. However, each time they jumped into the spring, they dirtied the water and wasted it by splashing this precious gift all over the ground.

Because of swimming this maiden developed an ear infection. The caretaker encouraged her to visit a local physician. When questioned, the maiden acknowledged that she and the caretaker regularly swam in the natural spring. The doctor advised her and the caretaker to stop swimming for their own health and for their town, which needed every drop of clean water. The caretaker and maiden refused to comply, since they truly enjoyed their sport. What the citizens of Spring City did not know could not hurt them, right?

Soon the doctor saw many patients who were infected with cholera. He identified drinking water from the spring as the source of their sickness. Therefore, required by law and in view of the citizens' health, this doctor alerted the mayor of Spring City to this couple's sport.

The mayor and city council members unanimously voted to fire the caretaker for his inappropriate behavior and harm inflicted on those in his care. Several in Spring City had befriended this caretaker and expressed sadness at his departure. The caretaker's friends devised a scheme to make the physician pay for his action.

Since many of the citizens in Spring City did not know the facts about the case, the local banker led a boycott against the physician. They publicly slandered his name by falsely claiming him to be unethical and unqualified. The lies did not take long to spread. Because of a failing practice, their physician moved his family to another town. The banker encouraged the citizens to remain loyal to the caretaker—one of their own.

Spring City exists today. Loyalty remains the city's motto; its spring remains unclean.

If the godly compromise with the wicked, it is like polluting a fountain or muddying a spring" (Prov. 25:26 NLT).

In the tale of Spring City, what role did correction play?

____

____

Broken relationships

Today we look at how Scripture provides correction for the believer. *Correction* describes the encouragement to follow the right way or the truthful, honest way. As Christ-followers this means that we obey God's will. Correction will include our confession of sin and a change of life direction.

Yet, before we look at how Scripture frequently corrects us, let us consider what would happen if we were to ignore God's correction through His inspired Word and conviction from the Holy Spirit.

In C. S. Lewis' book, *The Weight of Glory*, is a chapter entitled "The Inner Ring." Lewis addresses university students who are about to embark on their new careers. As they leave the shelter and disciplinary advice of their professors and parents, Lewis issues a warning on the ways of this world. He cautions against idolatry. Lewis writes:

"The prophecy I make is this. To nine out of ten of you the choice which could lead to scoundrelism will come, when it does come, in no very dramatic colours. Obviously bad men, obviously threatening or bribing, will almost certainly not appear. Over a drink or a cup of coffee, disguised as a triviality and sandwiched between two jokes, from the lips of a man, or woman, whom you have recently been getting to know rather better and whom you hope to know better still—just at the moment when you are most anxious not to appear crude, or naıf, or a prig—the hint will come. It will be the hint of something which is not quite in accordance with the technical rule of fair play . . . And then, if you are drawn in, next week it will be something a little further from the rules, and next year something further still, but all in the jolliest, friendliest spirit. It may end in a crash, a scandal, and penal servitude; it may end in millions, a peerage, and giving the prizes at your old school. But you will be a scoundrel."[1]

C. S. Lewis points out that whether you successfully hide your sin/our idol, you remain the same person. Even if sin's consequence has not impacted your family, the church, and your world, it will build a barrier between you and God. This is, I believe, the greatest consequence of ignoring correction.

The Bible says, *He who turns away his ear from listening to the law, even his prayer is an abomination* (Prov. 28:9 NASB). The Hebrew word for *listening* means "to hear, listen, obey."[2] This implies more than simply knowing truth. Listening requires obedience and not eloquence.

An *abomination* literally means *an idol*.[3] During Old Testament times the people of God regularly chose to worship idols made by people instead of worshiping "I AM" (Ex. 32). Their idol worship included horrific acts such as cutting their bodies (1 Kings 18:16-46), sacrificing their children (2 Kings 23:10), and immoral worship ceremonies (Num. 25). This was idol worship. God inspired the writer of this proverb to tell God's people that ignoring the law meant one chose to sin. As a result even their prayers were an abomination. This caution provides correction or discipline for us, too (Prov. 1:7).

Correction

We will study one specific passage in particular that I believe will help us understand how the Holy Spirit corrects Christians. Turn to Ephesians 5:1-20. Verses 1 and 2 provide a brief summary of how Christians are to follow Christ.

In these verses what characteristic of God does Paul emphasize?

____

Then verses 3-7 tell of the deeds that occur in darkness. In this passage we see a contrast between light and dark—a life lived controlled by sin or out of surrender to God.

Ephesians 5:8-10 explains how believers live as new creations. Please read this passage and then fill in the blanks below.

1) __________ *as children of light* (Eph 5:8).

2) __________, ______________, and ______________ characterize a life surrendered to God (Eph. 5:8).

3) *Figure out what will please Christ, and then* _____ _____ (Eph. 5:9 *The Message*).

Correction moves beyond rebuke; it seeks the restoration of a broken relationship and the furthering of your spiritual growth as a child of God.

Take time to mediate on this passage. Does the Holy Spirit bring to your mind an aspect of your life that needs to change? When God corrects you, run to Him, repent, and confess your sins. Take a moment to write down a prayer of surrender to God's loving correction.

____

____

____

If God shows you a specific step to help bring about this change, what is the step?

____

____

When do you plan to obey and make the change?

____

____

Today I want you to try a topical study of God's Word. During this lesson God may have brought to mind an area of your life in which you have sinned. Look up that topic in the concordance of your Bible. Read what God says about that issue. You may want to spend time memorizing a verse to help you fight temptation. Or, read James 4:1-12. This passage's theme is submission to God. Submission to God remains necessary when you fight temptation and combat evil.

May God bless the reading of His Word! Please listen with intent to obey.

Day 4 Health Bite

One of the most important choices individuals can make to promote good health is to be physically active. Often the most difficult part of an exercise program is being consistent. As a new year begins, jobs change, or the next season starts, everyone usually is motivated to become more fit and to change a diet. The problem is that the motivation does not continue for very long—schedules change or boredom or fatigue set in. Then the resolutions begin to falter.

Consistency can be the difference in a lifelong commitment. You wouldn't think of going more than a day without a shower, so don't go longer than a day without exercise. Maybe you need prayer support or a person who will hold you accountable. Do whatever is necessary to encourage yourself to get your daily exercise. Know that you are striving to become more fit to serve the Lord. *Whatever you are doing, work at it with enthusiasm, as to the Lord and not for people. . .. Serve the Lord Christ* (Col. 3:23-24 NET Bible).

Scheduling a time for your workout requires some thought and preparation. "When can I really schedule the time?" you may ask Early morning before the busy day begins, at noon during the lunch break, evenings and/or weekends are some suggested times. You will need at least a 30-minute block of time, three to five days a week.

Prepare a calendar with workout days noted with a red asterisk. Then log the actual workout once you complete it. Keeping records represents a good motivational method. You will enjoy charting your progress.

Challenge:: Walk 10 minutes.
Do 2 push-ups.
Do 10 crunches.

Week 1 - Day 5

The Last Days

Memory Verse:

All Scripture is God-breathed and is useful for teaching, rebuking, correcting and training in righteousness (2 Tim. 3:16 NIV).

Please turn to and read 2 Timothy 3.

2 Timothy 3:1-5 describes the last days. This time frame Paul terms *the last days* begins with the first century and continues until Christ's second coming.[1] Thus we can consider ourselves in the last days.

Do you see similarities between Paul's description and the world around you? If so, describe.

____

____

One phrase that sums up the message from this passage is found in verse 5: *Having a form of godliness but denying its power*. This phrase describes the people who do not follow Christ. Paul encourages Timothy to persevere when the world becomes more corrupt and destructive.

Paul also distinguishes between false teachers and the truth. *People will be lovers of themselves . . . lovers of pleasure rather than lovers of God-having a form of godliness but denying its power* (2 Tim. 3:2, 5). They may speak about Christ, but their lives do not include confession of their sin, surrender, or submission to God with a reliance on His strength to live differently. You likely noticed the theme of love. The central desire and passion in life of those to whom he describes is selfish and not focused on following Christ. It begins as a lack of love for God and manifests itself in all of their relationships.[2] They operate from a selfish nature. If they do receive a rebuke from Scripture, they reject it, because they worship an idol and not God.

Earlier this week we talked about how Scripture can provide more pleasure than food can. Also, the Bible exists as a vital means to help us remain faithful to Christ. The spiritual discipline of Scripture means that we are in God's Word on a daily basis so that He can teach, rebuke, correct, and now train us. We study Scripture for its sweetness and pleasure but also for survival.

Truth versus lies

Please read 2 Timothy 3:6-9.

Here Paul gives us examples of false teachers. In our information age verse 7 seems fitting. We often are on information overload; to which voice do we listen?

Can you think of a time in which your study of Scripture helped you identify a counterfeit message? If so, please write about this below.

____

____

This passage contains the only mention of Jannes and Jambres. However, Jewish tradition records them as magicians in Egypt who tried to mimic the signs from God (Ex. 7:11).[3]

People who oppose the truth will exist. We need to expect them. Therefore studying Scripture helps us to distinguish between true and false teaching.

Building endurance

In 2 Timothy 3:10-17 Paul gave a motivational speech. Yet, strangely enough, as Paul gives this charge, he tells Timothy to expect persecution. In fact, he says that everyone who follows Christ will be persecuted (2 Tim. 3:12).

Paul also gave two key points to Timothy that may help him persevere until the end.
1) The Lord will rescue us from the persecution, even if it ends in death, because He offers us eternal salvation. (2 Tim. 3:11 and Luke 12:1-12).
2) Consistency remains key (2 Tim. 3:14-15). The world will change, but Paul encourages Timothy to remain close to God. Practicing the spiritual discipline of studying Scripture helps us walk close to our Lord.

Training in righteousness

All Scripture is God-breathed and is useful for teaching, rebuking, correcting and training in righteousness (2 Tim. 3:16).

The final purpose of Scripture listed in this verse tells us to train in righteousness. We know that righteousness can occur only by faith in Christ (Rom. 4). However, God uses Scripture to train us as His children.[4]

Think about a child in your life. What role do you play or do you watch others play in this child's training? Write down the objective for training kids?

____

____

Our objective in training reaps immediate and long-term benefits. Here we see Paul encouraging Timothy to continue studying Scripture so he will remain faithful to Christ, identify false teaching, and experience God's comfort and faithfulness amidst persecution. After all, we have access to the inspired Word of God. These words have power.

The Bible says in Proverbs 22:6, *Train a child in the way he should go, and when he is old he will not turn from it.* Paul charges us, as children of God, to stick close to our Father. Know what He teaches, study His inspired Word, listen to His rebuke, follow His correction, and train as a child. May we all finish the race as faithful followers of Christ.

Today as you practice the spiritual discipline of studying God's Word, read 1 Peter 2:4-12. Fill in the following blanks.

What is the message about which Peter writes?

____

____

____

What characteristics does Paul use to describe this chosen people?

____

____

What difference does this make for those who believe the message about Jesus Christ?

____

____

Day 5 Health Bite

Change—how does the word impact you? What feelings does it evoke—anxiety, fear, excitement, apprehension? To be successful in any area of life, change is inevitable. Often the context in which we think about change affects how we respond to and deal with it. All of us arrive at a point in our lives at which we willingly are ready to commit and other times when we may be forced to change. Merely considering change can be a big step for some people who do not recognize that change is necessary or are overwhelmed by it.

At this moment in your life, what is your "stage of change" as it relates to improving your health? Refer to "Stages of Change" (page 190) in the appendix to evaluate whether you are ready to jump into a healthier lifestyle with two feet or just ready to test the waters!

Depending on your response, answer the following questions:

Ready: Fantastic! You are already on your way to making healthy changes!

Hesitant: Consider what would need to happen to move you to "ready"?

Resistant: Being resistant is OK. Think about when and if you may be ready to make changes. What would need to occur to allow you to start thinking about making "health" a greater priority?

We move in and out of the "stages of change" as we go through seasons of life. This is normal. In several weeks, months, or years, consider re-evaluating where you are.

Write out a list of pros and cons of making sacrifices that would allow wellness to be a priority in life.

PROS:	**CONS:**

"*Health is something positive, a joyful attitude toward life and cheerful acceptance of the responsibilities that life puts upon the individual*"—Henry E. Sigerist

Week 2 - Day 1

The Beginning

Memory Verse:

"This, then, is how you should pray. Our Father in heaven, hallowed be your name, your kingdom come, your will be done, on earth as it is in heaven. Give us today our daily bread. Forgive us our debts, as we also have forgiven our debtors. And lead us not into temptation but deliver us from the evil one" (Matt. 6:9-13).

For a moment let's review the context of Matthew 6, from which the above passage is taken. Matthew 6:5-6 provides a snapshot of individuals who pray as a way to promote their reputation as "spiritual" people—those worthy of recognition.

Christ taught that they have already received their reward, with their fleeting benefits gone in a flash. Yet pride blinded them from recognizing the one Whom they should have spotlighted—the one who had the power to answer their requests.

Matthew 6:9 says, *"This, then, is how you should pray. Our Father in heaven, hallowed be your name . . .."*

The subject: Father first

When you pray, *whom* does Matthew 6 instruct you to address?

____

In Matthew 6:9 Jesus clearly directs His followers as to how to begin. *Christ zooms in on the Father.*

The request

When you pray, *what* do you request? Below describe a typical "wish-list" that you offer to God in your prayers.

____

____

____

Matthew 6:9: *"Our Father in heaven, hallowed be your name . . .."*

Hallowed strikes me as such an ancient word—a word reserved for vacant cathedrals dotting the European countryside. These are noted for honoring history and saints but lacking in worship of God.

Quite the opposite is true, though. The real meaning of the word *hallowed* clues us in to the first request of the Lord's Prayer: that God would receive the recognition. We regard God as holy. This requires more than a fake smile and wordy prayer. It clarifies what lurks in the shadows of our hearts. For your prayers to honor God, view Him as set apart—above all—God, most high.

With the holiness of God in mind and our desire for His character expressed in the world, we may alter our current perspective on prayer. Instead of using it as a way to spotlight your exemplary practice of this spiritual discipline, use it as a time when—either alone or with others—you recognize the presence of God Who alone is worthy of praise. He is your focus.

Today take time to pray. Seek God alone today. Pray that God would receive the glory. Give Him the recognition for His work—past, present, and future. Then take time to offer confession, requests, and praise to God. As you pray the rest of the prayer, keep in mind the holiness of God.

If you would like to read a couple of beautiful prayers in which those crying out for God kept His holiness in mind, please read Isaiah 37 and Acts 4:23-31.

Day 1 Health Bite

Welcome to week 2! Hopefully last week you were able to identify reasons for placing health and wellness on your priority list. I challenge you to keep daily these reasons on the forefront of your mind to serve as a source of encouragement.

One of my favorite commercials for yogurt illustrates the impact of keeping our motivators "in sight"! The commercial shows a young woman hanging a yellow polka-dot bikini on her bedroom wall and gazing on it every day as a reminder to select yogurt as part of a healthy eating plan. This genius advertising has a lot of truth: if you keep right in front of you your reasons for changing your habits, you are more likely to be successful!

Use your personal motivation to encourage you to consistently make choices that will lead to meeting your vision for good health. You may want to consider spending part of your quiet time each day sharing with your Creator your thoughts and dreams for optimal health!

Food journaling can be an extremely effective means to promote self-awareness and accountability. As you continue your journey toward better health, you can use this information to evaluate changes you may need to make in your eating patterns or to identify the reasons you eat during the day.

How will you creatively remind yourself daily of your motivation for good health?

____

____

____

At least ________ days this week I will commit to journaling everything I eat and drink.

Goal-setting:

Write one positive and healthy change you plan to make in your eating habits.

____

____

____

* Refer to "SMART Goals" (page 188) in the appendix for a sample guide for goal-setting.

Week 2 - Day 2

Two Requests

Memory Verse:

"This, then, is how you should pray. Our Father in heaven, hallowed be your name, your kingdom come, your will be done, on earth as it is in heaven. Give us today our daily bread. Forgive us our debts, as we also have forgiven our debtors. And lead us not into temptation but believer us from the evil one" (Matt. 6:9-13).

The second section of the Lord's Prayer contains two requests. In today's lesson we'll study these.

Turn in your Bible to John 3 and read this chapter.

Thy Kingdom Come

The first request is contained in this verse: "***Thy kingdom come.*** *Thy will be done, On earth as it is in heaven*" [Emphasis mine] (Matt. 6:10 NASB).

What does God's kingdom look like? Below write down how Jesus, in John 3:1-12, describes the *kingdom of God.*

____

____

____

Here, we will focus on two key points from Jesus' teaching about the kingdom of God:
1) To enter the kingdom, you must receive salvation.
2) Members of the kingdom of God live a transformed life.

Kingdom of the saved

From the beginning of their conversation Jesus directs Nicodemus to the topic of salvation. Jesus states, *I tell you the truth, no one can enter the kingdom of God unless he is born of water and the Spirit* (John 3:5). *Born of water* is a reference to John the Baptist, who preaches a message of repentance and of the coming Messiah.[1] However, Jesus mentions a spiritual rebirth that surprises Nicodemus. The birth of *the spirit* refers to salvation by accepting salvation from Christ—a work of the Holy Spirit.

Look up John 3:14-15 and Numbers 21:1-9. What Old Testament reference does Jesus use for an explanation? What significance does this Old Testament event hold for Christians?

____

____

____

____

Turn in your Bibles to Matthew 5:17-20 and read this passage. According to Matthew 5:17-18, why is Jesus on earth?

____

____

As a Pharisee, Nicodemus follows the law as best he can and according to Scripture truly seeks to guide Israel. However, Jesus says, "*For I tell you that unless your righteousness surpasses that of the Pharisees and the teachers of the law, you will certainly not enter the kingdom of heaven*" (Matt. 5:20). Nicodemus needs a Savior, too.

Living by the Truth

Second, this passage addresses transformation (John 3:16-21). Here we find one of the most famous verses—John 3:16. Yet, by further reading, this passage distinguishes between those who enter God's kingdom and those who reject His salvation.

List distinguishing characteristics of those who accept Christ's message.

____

____

____

____

Friend of the Bridegroom

John the Baptist prepares the way for Christ. He calls all to repentance and points to the Messiah. In John 3, we see John's disciples frustrated that Jesus is developing a larger following. John 3:27-30 gives John the Baptist's reply. He focuses on his assignment and is never deterred.

As Christians we have a very similar calling. Our difference rests in the fact we know Jesus died, rose again, and will return to reign here on the earth (Acts 18:18-28).

Thy Will Be Done

The second half of this request asks that God's will be done. The prayer asks, "***Thy will be done, On earth as it is in heaven***" [emphasis mine] (Matt. 6:10 NASB).

John the Baptist again represents a wonderful example for us. He has the right perspective of purpose and prominence.

Purpose relates to a job description. John the Baptist fulfills his calling of a messenger preparing the way for the Messiah (Matt. 11:10). John humbly serves even when the crowds fade. When you accomplish God's will, intentionally place prominence on Christ.

The Bridegroom

At this time, those in my social circle have busied themselves preparing for a wedding. As the maid of honor, I get to partake in all of the wedding festivities and preparations. As I study this passage, I'm reminded of Elizabeth and Robert (not their real names)—the bride and groom in the wedding in which I'm participating. They work as Bible translators. She is a linguist and he a computer programmer.

From the time she was in middle school, Elizabeth knew God called her into missions. During high school God began to lead her toward translation. Early on Elizabeth became known for her intelligence. Teachers suggested she study engineering or medicine. But by that time, she knew her role in the kingdom involved missions—specifically Bible translation. She consistently readied herself for that call.

Robert grew up and became a successful computer programmer. After he traveled on a short-term mission trip, he knew God led him to go into missions. He then made plans to sell his possessions and head to Texas for training in translation.

Robert and Elizabeth met at the Wycliff training center in Texas. The first time Elizabeth introduced me to Robert, they stated that they both loved America but felt compelled by the Lord to go overseas and spread the gospel.

They represent modern-day examples of John the Baptist. As translators they will serve one people group for most, if not all, of their lives. Translators often serve behind the scenes as they work diligently to develop a written language and then translate the Bible, God's inspired Word, for the first time into that language. What a blessing to bring a story of love, grace, salvation, and repentance to a people who have never heard God's truth before!

John said, "*The bride belongs to the bridegroom. The friend who attends the bridegroom waits and listens for him, and is full of joy when he hears the bridegroom's voice. That joy is mine, and it is now complete. He must become greater and I must become less*" (John 3:29-30).

God has designed a unique place for all His children to serve in His kingdom. But the question of **purpose** and **prominence** remains. We all have a calling to share the hope we have in Christ. Will you follow faithfully?

Take a moment to pray for God's kingdom to come and for His will to be done. In the space below write out your prayer.

____

____

____

____

____

____

Read a story of two who faithfully sought God's kingdom and will. In Esther 4 read about Queen Esther. In Acts 20-21 read about Paul. Take time for prayer. Make sure you spend time asking that God's kingdom and will be done on the earth now.

Day 2 Health Bite

You have just read about guidelines that help us learn how to pray. We also have some exercise guidelines to help us become more physically fit.

The workout has three parts. The **warmup** can include stretching and light activity to prepare the body for more intense work. The **conditioning bout** (main workout) is the activity itself. It could be walking, jogging, cycling, swimming, etc. During this segment the heart rate needs to be elevated. The length of time can be extended as your level of fitness improves. The **cool-down** consists of slowing down but not stopping. Do some additional stretching while the body is warm and the heart rate begins to return to normal.

Assume that health improvement is forever. *We will not sit down until he comes*, says 1 Samuel 16:11 (The Message). As Christians our job here on earth is to expand the kingdom of God through evangelism, Bible study, and the discipleship of others. Fulfilling the Lord's commission requires that we be in the best shape possible. We have a lot of work to do before the Lord's return, so let's get ready to do it!

Challenge: Progress through a workout while you note the three segments:

- Warm up for 3 minutes, walk purposefully for 9 minutes, and then cool down for 3 minutes.
- Do 4 push-ups.
- Do 15 crunches.

Week 2 - Day 3

Oscar, the Office Bird

Memory Verse:

"This, then, is how you should pray. Our Father in heaven, hallowed be your name, your kingdom come, your will be done, on earth as it is in heaven. Give us today our daily bread. Forgive us our debts, as we also have forgiven our debtors. And lead us not into temptation but deliver us from the evil one" (Matt. 6:9-13).

During college I was a typical college student involved in classes, work, and averaging four extracurricular organizations a year. I constantly faced stress. One week in particular, I remember feeling unusually overwhelmed.

I worked part-time at our student-life center in the nutrition-education program. My job as student educator was to promote healthy lifestyles on campus. One day that week, I reached our office on the third floor and found a bird flying around the track. *What in the world is a bird doing in the gym?* I wondered. I opened the office door, turned on the lights, and went to work.

Ever so quietly and cautiously, in flew the bird. I quickly closed the door behind him and called the maintenance team to pick up our gym's newest visitor. As I worked on the computer and prepared a booth for our next health fair, I heard this bird check out our office.

This random bird definitely brought humor to my day, so I decided to name him *Oscar.* We talked about everything on my plate and my rising stress level. He was a very good listener, so we bonded.

For the most part he behaved well, except when a student stopped by to pick up some nutrition information and Oscar perched on our flyer rack or when he jumped around on the poster boards we had been preparing for the fair.

After a few hours, I left to go to class. The bird was still in our office waiting for someone to take him home. Once I was outside, I called my Mom and told her about Oscar; in addition, I asked that she pray for me just to survive the busy day. My mom is my prayer warrior. Before I hung up the phone, my mom said, "God sent you a sparrow." "What?" I asked. She repeated, "Literally, God sent you a sparrow. God is watching over you, so don't worry."

The rest of the day I kept thinking, *God you really are amazing! You just used a bird in a gym to remind me that You are in control and will provide for what I need today. Thanks!* I was reminded of the verse, *Look at the birds of the air; they do not sow or reap or store away in barns, and yet your heavenly Father feeds them. Are you not much more valuable than they? Who of you by worrying can add a single hour to his life?* (Matt. 6:26-27).

Prayer for provision

Read Matthew 6:25-34. In the space below please write a characteristic of God you see illustrated in this passage.

____

____

____

____

Five times in Matthew 6:25-34 Jesus mentions anxiety. Three of the times He specifically states, "*Do not be anxious.*" He then gives two reasons why:

1) Look at creation and see that your Creator takes care of all things, including you (vv. 26 and 28-30).
2) Anxiety has no benefit (vv. 27 and 34).

One of my closest friends since college is another dietitian named Stephanie. While we were at Baylor, we studied together in nutrition and science classes, worked together at the student-life center, were involved in several of the same extracurricular activities, and occasionally attended each other's churches.

Stephanie and I started praying together before work. We would pray for God's direction and His glorification in and through us. Stephanie was a wonderful encouragement during stressful times as well. When we felt like complaining, we would remind each other that stressing out only wasted time.

I encourage you this week to meet with an accountability partner and specifically spend time in prayer together. Maybe take a prayer walk outside and praise God for his creativity and provision.

Why should I pray?

Recently I spoke with a Christian friend who really wanted to know why she should pray. Her logic, "If God is sovereign and all-knowing, why does He want me to ask

Him? It seems like a waste of time."

Honestly, I understand where she is coming from. I've had times in my life in which I don't seem to get a response from God, so I become very frustrated with my prayer life. Prayer has always been one of the weaker areas of my relationship with God.

But after I read on prayer and discussed this with mentors, I discovered some words of wisdom that changed my life. I would like to share these with you.

First, investigate "why" you pray. This is the second pitfall of prayer that Jesus mentions in Matthew 6:5-8. Prayer exists as a key communication vehicle with God. But He cautions against praying in public when you do not pray in private. Take a moment—if you are struggling with motivation to pray, evaluate "why" and "where" you pray. Do you only pray at church or at meals with other believers? What about on a daily basis—alone, when no one sees you?

God wants us to pray privately and corporately; we see this in Matthew 6:5-8. If you read most commentaries on the Lord's Prayer, most quickly point out the use of plural pronouns, such as "*Our Father*". We are expected to pray corporately. But just as Scripture reading indicates, if you do not pray on a daily basis alone with God, then your relationship most likely is stagnant. Think of it as giving God a call on your cell phone. Don't just send Him a text message and turn off your phone.

Our communication with God should be open, like Adam and Eve had in the garden before the fall. If not, just like Adam and Eve, sometimes sin may be the reason that we limit our prayer time.

Richard Foster, a well-respected author on spiritual disciplines, wrote in *Celebration of Discipline*, "To pray is to change. Prayer is the central avenue God uses to transform us. If we are unwilling to change, we will abandon prayer as a noticeable characteristic of our lives."[1]

If you have abandoned prayer, you may have not surrendered completely to God's Lordship. Evaluate your life to see if you have allowed sin to have a foothold.

Many mentors have told me that Christians are expected to pray. They referenced me to Paul's writings on how a Christian is to act. First Thessalonians 5:16-18 (NASB) says, *Rejoice always; pray without ceasing; in everything give thanks; for this is God's will for you in Christ Jesus.*"

Today in your quiet time, look at your calendar. Schedule a time to pray. Consider going to your church's prayer room to help you prioritize your time with God. Also, find a friend with whom you can schedule a time to walk or get coffee or hot

tea together. Catch up on life, take time to thank God for His daily provision, and then pray for each other.

Spend time reading Scripture. If you would like a little direction, read James 5:13-20. *Taste and see that the Lord is good; blessed is the man who takes refuge in him. Fear the Lord, you his saints, for those who fear him lack nothing. The lions may grow weak and hungry, but those who seek the Lord lack no good thing* (Ps. 34:8-10).

Day 3 Health Bite

In both the Old and New Testaments, the Lord provides food for His people when they are in need. Our current culture is a land of "plenty" and "excess". This makes abusing this luxury through overindulgence easy. God created us to eat throughout the day for energy and nourishment. Our metabolism is what turns fuel (food) into energy. For optimal energy and weight-control the act of eating helps keep our metabolism revved up!

Many examples in the Bible demonstrate God's provision of appropriate food choices for His children. Carbohydrates are necessary for energy. Like a car needs gas, we will not function appropriately without them! Protein sources help maintain lean muscle mass and promote a healthy immune system. Fat sources regulate hormones and can assist with disease prevention. The body requires a longer time to break down protein and fat (compared with carbs); this causes one to feel dissatisfied and full.

If we fail to balance our macronutrients (protein, carbohydrates, and fat) throughout the day, our appetites and energy are influenced. Several times this week, try using the model below—the "Idaho Plate Method".[1] Developed by the University of Idaho, it is a visual guide for eating healthy—to balance your plate. This method recommends filling half of your plate with vegetables, one-fourth with a starch, and one-fourth with meat or other protein source. Take time to thank the Lord for the provision of food. How might this mindful act of thanks impact how you view and approach the food?

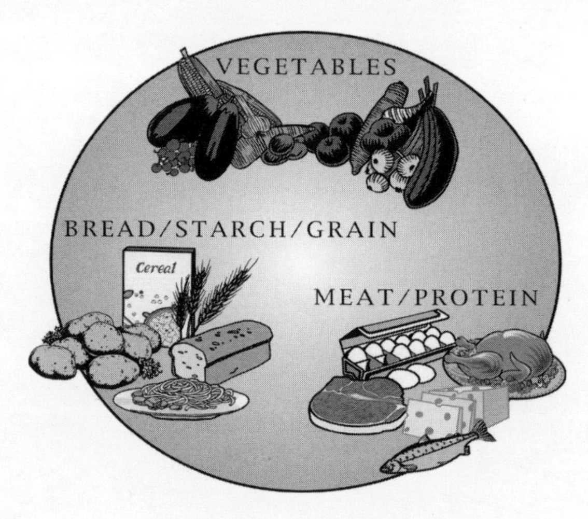

Goals:

I will limit my protein portion to three to four ounces at meal times (lunch/dinner) ____ days this week.

I will include vegetables at dinner at least _______ times this week.

I will use the "Plate Method" concept at least ______ times this week. Make a point to thank the Lord for the food you enjoy!

Week 2 - Day 4

The Pastor's Daughter

Memory Verse:

"This, then, is how you should pray. Our Father in heaven, hallowed be your name, your kingdom come, your will be done, on earth as it is in heaven. Give us today our daily bread. Forgive us our debts, as we also have forgiven our debtors. And lead us not into temptation but deliver us from the evil one" (Matt. 6:9-13).

"China for 500," I said.

"This missionary baked cookies to meet her neighbors," Mrs. Ruby stated.

"Who is Lottie Moon?" I quickly responded.

"Correct; 500 hundred points for . . . Samantha." Mrs. Ruby said, as she added 500 points to my friend's score.

"No!" I said with emphasis. "I earned those points."

"Stephanie, I already told you. You're the pastor's daughter. This isn't fair to the others," she responded with exasperation.

"But we only have Girls in Action on Wednesdays. She already got her points," I added.

"And . . . " Mrs. Ruby turned her back to me . . .. "Anne, what category do you want?"

I wanted to cry and scream in anger all at the same time. But no, I was in fifth grade and had to hatch up a plan. This was the third week Mrs. Ruby gave my points away. I had warned her last week; she left me no other alternative. (By the way, I've changed the real names of all the people in this story.)

So I pushed my chair back from the table, spun around, and headed for the door. Mrs. Ruby saw me get up. "Stephanie, if you leave, you will get in *so* much trouble when you get home!"

"No, I won't," I muttered back.

"When your parents pick you up and you are not here, then you will get in trouble for skipping" she remarked.

"No, I am going to stand outside the doorway and tell them that you never give me my points because I'm the pastor's daughter!"

I stood right outside the classroom with my arms crossed, teeth clenched, and eyebrows hunched in anger.

Anger management

That night, before my parents stopped by for me, another teacher found me. After confirming the accuracy of the circumstance, the teacher removed me from Mrs. Ruby's guidance. My parents and other leaders confronted a couple of women besides Mrs. Ruby who chose to treat me in a similar manner. When they were approached, these women refused to change. I remember other adults making apologizes for them. I accepted these and acted as if all was well.

I forgave as a fifth-grader could. As a new believer I knew what the Bible taught and tried my best to obey.

These events may seem miniscule. A kid didn't get stickers or awards. Maybe he or she got chewed out for something the person did not do. So what? But to a fifth-grader a huge injustice occurred; before I even reached middle-school age, I had planted a seed of bitterness in my heart toward the church.

Forgiveness

Today we will study forgiveness. I believe this message hits at the core of many hearts.

Matthew 6:12 and 14-15 says, "*Forgive us our debts, as we also have forgiven our debtors . . .. For if you forgive men when they sin against you, your heavenly Father will also forgive you. But if you do not forgive men their sins, your Father will not forgive your sins.*"

Faith first

Matthew 6:12 and 14-15 could easily lead to a misunderstanding, so I issue this word of caution. Before you plunge into this passage on forgiveness, please read Ephesians 2:1-10. These verses help set the foundation of our study today. These verses from

Ephesians highlight two points. **First, our salvation is a gift from God**. Nothing we do can earn salvation. **Second, because we have accepted this salvation, we have chosen a new way of life**. By God's grace we received salvation; by grace we act differently.

Forgiveness guidelines

Now turn back to Matthew 6—our primary passage this week—to read the Lord's Prayer. Please take a moment and summarize Matthew 6:12 in your own words. Specifically think about and comment on the phrase *as we also.*

____

____

____

A debt you could not repay

Please turn to and read Matthew 18:21-35.

In Matthew 18:21, what does Peter really want to know? We know Peter already chooses an overly generous number of times to forgive others. Typically the Jewish rabbis teach people they can stop forgiving after three offenses.[2] Basically Peter wants to know when he could stop the kindness and forgiveness. Jesus responds *I tell you, not seven times, but seventy-seven times* (Matt. 18:22). From His response we can see God wants forgiveness to become a habit for His followers.

The parable tells us of the first man who owes 10,000 talents. He has a debt for millions of dollars—an amount he simply cannot pay.[2] Please write a summary of this man's view about forgiveness—both the forgiveness he receives and why he refuses to give it.

____

____

____

Now summarize the master's view of forgiveness. Why does he demand that this man forgive a fellow servant?

____

____

The Bible says, "*Shouldn't you have had mercy on your fellow servant just as I had on you?*" (Matt. 18:33). The master obviously symbolizes God (v. 35). As Christians we claim to have accepted God's forgiveness. By accepting God's forgiveness and grace we realize the punishment we deserve for our sin.

Yet sometimes along the road of the Christian life, we choose not to forgive. Did we forget what happened when God forgave all of our sins, wiped away our punishment, and then pronounced us His children? He did not have to do this! Just like the master does in Matthew 18, God takes pity on us and pays the price Himself. He cancels our debt.

God's grace changes our lives. First, it gives us freedom to live debt-free. Second, we have the ability and expectation to show God's grace to others. Automatically forgiving others and giving grace may not seem natural. Yet, for a Christian it becomes a way of life.

Baggage

When I was a young adult, in my prayer life God challenged me about forgiveness, so I often approach God confessing sin, repenting, and asking forgiveness. Matthew 6 taught me to pray, "Lord, as I forgive others, please forgive me." After I meditated on this passage and evaluated my life, I realized one place I needed to forgive. This emotional baggage had existed since elementary school; I did not want to pop open the trunk.

About this time God began placing a desire in my heart to enter the ministry. When I was a sixth-grader, God tugged on my heart for the first time to serve Him in ministry. But of course, I had fresh wounds. They seemed to be the perfect reason that ministry and I did not belong together.

Who is your daddy?

Sorting through my emotional baggage and my lack of forgiveness brought up many childhood memories. I wondered why as a fifth-grader I first began to talk back. I got the boldness from an understanding of my new faith in Christ and teaching from my dad.

My parents spent time discipling my brother and me. My dad taught that he wanted us to follow the guidelines of our heavenly Father. He would say, "I will never ask you to do something because I am a pastor. I will ask you to behave a certain way because you follow Christ."

Jesus told us in John 15:20, "*Remember the words I spoke to you: 'No servant is greater than his master.' If they persecuted me, they will persecute you also. If they obeyed my teaching, they will obey yours also.*'"

When I was a child, I grew to expect mistreatment from some people because of who my dad was. It went with the territory. I never got upset at my parents nor wanted us to change from being a ministerial family. My dad remains the godliest guy I know; I have observed him for my whole life, so I should know.

As an adult I realized that all believers will receive persecution because we follow Christ. The beautiful thing is that along with the reason for persecution, a means to relate to the persecutor goes with it. By faith in Christ we become the children of God; as children of God we follow His example by giving grace and forgiveness to others. We can honestly pray, "*Forgive us our debts, as we also have forgiven our debtors*" (Matt. 6:12).

What about you? Did God remind you of a person you need to forgive?

Please read Ephesians 4:17-5:2. As you read it, meditate on each verse and pray.

Day 4 Health Bite

We learned today how an understanding of forgiveness results in our forgiveness of others. Love toward others takes effort. [Love] *bears all things, believes all things, hopes all things, endures all things (*1 Cor. 13:7 NASB). Love is a choice. So is exercise.

The Lord didn't burden us with work. He blessed us with it. But the Lord in His infinite wisdom blessed us with work so that we could enjoy the fruit of our labor and the satisfaction that accompanies the toil of our efforts.

Our workouts can be likewise—not a burden but a true blessing. When we work out, the body improves and becomes stronger. We are more energized; that is a true blessing.

Fitness is the capability of the heart, blood vessels, lungs, and muscles to function at optimal efficiency. This level is needed to go through our busy daily routines. To develop and maintain fitness requires a vigorous effort by all the body systems. Fitness has been divided into four components. During the workout, consider each one.

1. Cardiorespiratory (*cardio* for short) is the aerobic part of the workout. The heart rate must be elevated for at least 20-30 minutes.
2. Strength and muscular endurance is the part of the workout in which weights or other forms of resistance are used. Using weights or our own body weight to create a resistance puts an extra load on the muscle. When this is repeated over time, the muscle group becomes stronger to accommodate the new workload.
3. Flexibility is the ability to move at the joints. Good flexibility can reduce the risk of injury to the connective tissue. Some activities, such as gymnastics and dance, require greater flexibility. Flexibility can be improved through systematic stretching.
4. Body composition is the relationship of the lean muscle tissue to that of the fat tissue. This relationship can change with a consistent workout when we decrease the fat stores and increase the muscle mass.

Challenge: Walk for 20 minutes
Do 4 push-ups
Do 15 crunches

Week 2 - Day 5

Lead Us Not into Temptation

Memory Verse:

"This, then, is how you should pray. Our Father in heaven, hallowed be your name, your kingdom come, your will be done, on earth as it is in heaven. Give us today our daily bread. Forgive us our debts, as we also have forgiven our debtors. And lead us not into temptation but deliver us from the evil one" (Matt. 6:9-13).

Jesus tells His followers to pray that they will not fall into temptation (Matt. 6:13). In the Garden of Gethsemane he repeats this charge to His disciples (Mark 14:38).

When it teaches on *temptation,* the Bible refers to one of two different definitions. Temptation is "any attempt to entice or tempt into evil; a testing which aims at an ultimate spiritual good."[1]

1. Enticement

For the first definition, please turn to and read James 1:13-15. After you read this, please write down the source of our temptation.

For more information on the wickedness of the human heart, read Jeremiah 17:1-10.

James 4:1-10 gives us a proved way to avoid temptation. James 4:7 says when you are tempted, you are to *Submit yourselves, then, to God. Resist the devil, and he will flee from you.*

2. Test of growth

The second type of temptation refers to a temptation/discipline that God allows so that we will grow into mature followers of Christ.

Please read Hebrews 12:1-13. Based on Hebrews 12 below write a summary describing the Lord's discipline.

____

____

____

____

Remember what the Bible says: *No discipline seems pleasant at the time but painful. Later on, however, it produces a harvest of righteousness and peace for those who have been trained by it* (Heb. 12:11).

Personal evaluation

1. Take a moment and think about the first definition of *temptation.* How do you respond when you are tempted by your own evil desires? Below write your plan of resisting temptation the next time it raises its ugly head.

____

____

____

2. Now consider the second definition of *temptation.* Have you ever had a time in your life in which you were under the Lord's discipline and you believe He used this to strengthen your faith and relationship with Him? Below please write about that experience.

____

____

____

The Bible says "*And do not lead us into temptation, but deliver us from evil.* [For Thine is the kingdom, and the power, and the glory, forever. Amen] (Matt. 6:13 Holman).

We will face temptation. However, we serve the Lord Almighty. He holds supreme authority and power over all. When we submit to Him, He can and will deliver us from evil.

Spend time in prayer and Scripture reading; you may want to read John 15 and 16 as encouragement to resist temptation. This weekend, please consider reading Revelation 7 and Daniel 6; these chapters describe how God saves His people.

"I have told you these things, so that in me you may have peace. In this world you will have trouble. But take heart! I have overcome the world" (John 16:33).

Day 5 Health Bite

"Ohhh . . . that strawberry cheesecake tasted so divine! Instead of the 'three-bite limit', I ate the entire ____ pound serving!"

Often clients arrive at the office "confessing" their food temptations and punishing themselves over lack of control and overindulging in less-than-healthy foods. How many of you view high-fat, high-sugar, or high-carb foods as the "enemy"? I challenge you to stop and consider making peace with these "enemies".

I am sure you have heard that "all food can fit"—do you believe it? Some foods we should eat more often and others less often, but we have no food we should completely give up. Consider committing to nutrient-dense foods at least 85 percent of the time.

If you tend to overindulge in less-healthy foods, what attracts you to these foods? Do they taste better? Did you grow up with these foods and have trouble breaking the habit? Do these foods pop into your day when you are stressed, bored, or feeling sad? Consider three strategies to limit the "sometimes food."

1. Find ways to limit but not completely avoid these foods (unless it is a "trigger food" and you have no control when you eat it.) "Diets" start and stop. Hopefully you aspire to commit to a lifestyle change.
2. Search for palatable substitutions to your high-fat favorites. (If you have a sweet tooth, consider lower-calorie alternatives. If you love your fried favorites, consider experimenting in the kitchen with new cooking styles.)
3. Give yourself grace. Don't beat yourself up over not meeting your nutrition goals. Look forward, not backward. Move on with optimism to the next meal. Select healthier choices.

Goals to avoid temptation:

• I will eat every three to four hours. (Consider making a meal schedule.)

• I will limit fried food/sweets to _______ times this week.

• I will evaluate my "fluid calories". Am I limiting beverages that are high in sugar?

What are two to three goals toward which I can move in the week ahead?

____

____

____

Week 3 - Day 1

King Uzziah

Memory Verse:

"'Yet a time is coming and has now come when true worshipers will worship the Father in spirit and truth, for they are the kind of worshipers the Father seeks. God is spirit, and his worshipers must worship in spirit and in truth.' The woman said, 'I know that Messiah' (called Christ) 'is coming. When he comes, he will explain everything to us.' Then Jesus declared, 'I who speak to you am he'"
(John 4:23-26).

In the year of King Uzziah's death (Isaiah 6:1a NASB). This short, dense phrase explains the climate of the times. Isaiah the prophet serves God under the reign of several kings, one of whom is King Uzziah. Uzziah goes down in history as a well-loved and successful king of Judah. He initially seeks God. God grants him both economic and military accomplishments. However, Uzziah allows pride to seep into his life. This leads to his downfall.

But when he became strong, his heart was so proud that he acted corruptly, and he was unfaithful to the Lord his God, for he entered the temple of the Lord to burn incense on the altar of incense (2 Chron. 26:16 NASB). The priests know that King Uzziah acts in disobedience to God's instructions for worship; they confront him in the temple (2 Chron. 26:17-18 and Num. 16:40). Yet King Uzziah only responds with anger; his reaction to this confrontation further highlights his personal idolatry. At that moment, the Lord afflicts him with leprosy (2 Chron. 26:19). King Uzziah leaves the temple and spends the rest of his life in isolation.

Hope, pride, and worship

Isaiah 6 recounts the story of this prophet's encounter with God Almighty. What is the significance of Isaiah 6:1a for worship? Scripture highlights several points that we can apply to our lives.

The climate of the times in Judah and the Western world today holds numerous similarities.

1) For starters we can both claim economic success.
2) Both can claim military power.
3) Both also can claim sinful, prideful lives.

Our pride in our own abilities and resources can directly interfere with worship. For just like Uzziah, unless God strips away our hope and pride in anything other than Himself, our acts of worship serve as a cheap veil for our idolatry.

A.W. Tozer wrote a book called *Whatever Happened to Worship*? Referring to Isaiah 6 he says, "I tell you again that God has saved us to be worshipers. May God show us a vision of ourselves that will disvalue us to the point of total devaluation. From there He can raise us up to worship Him and to praise Him and to witness."[1]

Isaiah started telling about his encounter with God by stating a monumental event in Judah—the death of King Uzziah. The people of Judah possibly questioned their confidence in the future; maybe the recent news probably shattered their previously stable world.

My parents' generation can tell us how the unexpected death of President Kennedy shocked their generation. September 11 and Hurricane Katrina rattled mine. During these moments, as a nation people sought God. We flooded into churches and worshiped Him together.

This week we will study the spiritual discipline of worship. But first take a moment to assess your life. Often good things in our lives can turn into idols and inhibit our worship.

So as we begin this look at worship, I encourage you to take a moment and think about in what you have hope. I pray your hope of salvation lies in Christ (Heb. 6:16-20).

Please answer these questions:
In the past how have you responded when life went amuck?

____

____

____

____

____

____

____

What is the climate of our times?

____

____

In *The Knowledge of the Holy*, A.W. Tozer wrote, "This loss of the concept of majesty has come just when the forces of religion are making dramatic gains and the churches are more prosperous than at any time within the past several hundred years. But the alarming thing is that our gains are mostly external and our losses are wholly internal; and since it is the quality of our religion that is affected by internal conditions, it may be that our supposed gains are but losses spread over a wider field."

He continued, "The only way to recoup our spiritual losses is to go back to the cause of them and make such corrections as the truth warrants. The decline of the knowledge of the holy has brought on our troubles. A rediscovery of the majesty of God will go a long way toward curing them. It is impossible to keep our moral practices sound and our inward attitudes right while our idea of God is erroneous or inadequate. If we would bring back spiritual power to our lives, we must begin to think of God more nearly as He is."[2]

Overweight and malnourished

Around the world we have noticed a phenomenon termed *overweight and malnourished.* This concept may seem counter-intuitive. How can someone be classified as *malnourished* if the person is overweight? *Malnourishment* refers to more than an individual's body weight. It includes his or her protein and nutrient stores.

As a dietitian I know that the individual habitually consumes a large volume of high-calorie foods that provides minimal protein and nutrients—low-nutrient density. I also may make the assumption that this person rarely exercises.

The solution: cut back on excessive calories that do not have protein, vitamins, and minerals. The recommendation: eat a balanced diet of protein, carbohydrates, and fat and incorporate at least five to nine fruits and vegetables a day and exercise. You easily could find this information on the Internet. So why do people go to meet with a dietitian or exercise specialist? For application. Knowledge alone does not solve the problem.

Reading books about worship do not automatically turn you into a true worshiper who continues to learn more about God and becomes more committed to following Christ. The problem lies in lack of application. Here we find the purpose of practicing the spiritual discipline of worship.

Spiritual nourishment

When we allow our stability and strength to rest in anything other than God, then we easily can become malnourished. Your idols may feed you well. The consequence of worshiping them provides plenty of enjoyment, but just like your physical state you become spiritually malnourished because your pursuits and goals are empty and meaningless. Only true worship nourishes our spiritual health.

Take a moment and reflect on your spiritual health. When I go to the doctor for my wellness checkup, the people there take lab specimens. I either get a phone call, email, or letter with their summary of my lab values.

If the Great Physician were to look at your spiritual health, what do you think He would include in the summary?

____

____

____

Take your Bible and spend some time studying God's Word. Today we looked at Judah as Isaiah notes the end of a prosperous reign. King Solomon, another famous king, wrote the book of Ecclesiastes. Solomon pursues everything the world offers and finds that without God, all is meaningless. I encourage you to read Ecclesiastes 1-2 and meditate on Isaiah 6:1.

Scripture provides examples for us. Yet history repeats itself. Write about a time in which your world shook.

____

____

To whom or to what did you run?

____

Based on the Bible was this a wise choice?

____

If not, what do you plan to change next time?

____

____

____

____

Day 1 Health Bite

Water—we have all heard that drinking it will keep us healthy. "Eight glasses of water a day" often is the general rule health professionals give; however this may not be sufficient for everyone. The recommendation for water intake varies and is based on a person's environment, weight, and exercise habits. An estimated 75 percent of Americans suffer from mild chronic dehydration, which may result in fuzzy short-term memory, difficulty focusing, or exhaustion.

Next to air, water is essential for human survival. The human body is 55 to 70 percent water. A mere two-percent drop in your body's water supply can trigger signs of dehydration. Your body is unable to replenish itself; all cell and organ functions depend on it doing so. Water serves as a lubricant, regulates body temperature, alleviates constipation, and regulates metabolism; therefore it can help boost metabolism and aid in disease prevention!

Drink up!

- Set reminders on your watch, computer, or pager!
- Keep a pitcher, jug, or water bottle within reach throughout the day.
- Avoid becoming thirsty. By that point you are already dehydrated!
- Limit caffeinate-containing beverages that fail to re-hydrate you. Try using lemon, lime, orange, or cucumber to make water more appealing!

Take a moment to thank God for the unique design of the human body. Consider how drinking water may be a way to honor your body and the One who created you!

On average how much water do I drink each day? ____________________________

GOAL: I will drink _______ounces at least ________ times a week this week.

My plan to accomplish this goal:

____

____

____

____

One of the best indicators of dehydration is the color of your urine. If it is pale yellow to clear in color, you are doing great! If not, drink up!

Week 3 - Day 2

Wet, Wind, and Worship

Memory Verse:

"'Yet a time is coming and has now come when true worshipers will worship the Father in spirit and truth, for they are the kind of worshipers the Father seeks. God is spirit, and his worshipers must worship in spirit and in truth.' The woman said, 'I know that Messiah' (called Christ) 'is coming. When he comes, he will explain everything to us.' Then Jesus declared, 'I who speak to you am he'"
(John 4:23-26).

One spring weekend I planned time to spend with God and sort through a few issues. I wanted to get away from the chaos of life that I encountered at college. So I went home. After the short, two-hour drive I grabbed my Bible and went out to the wood fort in the back yard, where my brother and I played when we were children. I grew up in a small suburb of Dallas. Where we live looks like the country. Behind our back yard another family owns a large plot of land on which the owners keep horses and grow wildflowers in the spring. Beyond lies an undeveloped flood plain.

That day the clouds hovered overhead as though they were a gray shadow. At the top of the fort I felt a cool breeze that zipped around me. I shook down to my bones. I stood silent as I looked at the land beyond. We were in the midst of bluebonnet season. The bluebonnets had grown so thick that they looked as though they formed a blue lake with gentle waves rippling with the wind.

The clouds suddenly dropped a gentle rain. I stood for a minute and took in the beauty of creation. Then I crouched down in the corner of the fort and laid out my Bible on the floor.

On the drive home from college I had created a mental agenda of things to bring before the Lord. But as I heard the wind whistle over the rough, wooden fort planks, I knew my agenda would wait. I didn't like to stand for long exposed to a gentle spring shower. Yet, God, the Creator allows us in His presence. *Amazing*. I had gone home to talk business with God, but the truth was, I needed to worship Him.

Please take a worship break and read Ephesians 2:11-22. Meditate on this passage. Spend time praising and thanking Christ for the undeserved gift He offers and all of the benefits that go with it.

Creator versus created

Please open your Bibles to Romans 1:20. This verse tells how creation testifies to God the Creator. Paul states that by creation all humankind can see evidence of Divinity. Romans 1:25 NASB says, *For they exchanged the truth of God for a lie, and worshiped and served the creature rather than the Creator, who is blessed forever. Amen.* But throughout history people have chosen to worship the temporary, created things instead of the Eternal Creator.

Louie Giglio writes in *The Air I Breathe,* "Should you for some reason choose not to give God what He desires, you'll worship anyway—simply exchanging the Creator for something He has created."[1] Romans 1 reminds us how creation can inspire worship of the Creator—we must recognize *Who* we worship.

Yesterday we studied Isaiah 6:1; today we continue in Isaiah 6. Unlike Isaiah and John (Rev. 4) we should probably count on seeing the throne room of God only when we die. So what do we do now while we're still on earth? Scripture teaches us how to worship.

The throne of God

Open your Bible to and read Isaiah 6:2-4 and Revelation 4:1-11. Scripture tells that God sits on a throne. The throne symbolizes authority, royalty, and power.

God exists above all; He alone is worthy of worship. Isaiah 6:1 says He is lofty and exalted. Revelation 4:10-11 says God is exalted above all and receives the praise and adoration from His creation.

Read Isaiah 6:3 and Revelation 4:8. Take a moment to reflect on the Holiness of God. In the phrase *Holy, Holy, Holy*, the repetition of the word shows importance besides describing God as completely holy.

How would you define *holiness*? Below please write your definition.

____

____

____

The New Merriam Webster Dictionary defines *holy* as: 1) worthy of absolute devotion, 2) sacred, and 3) having a divine quality.[2]

Worship defines not only attending a service but the devotion of our lives. This spills out into our thoughts, emotions, and actions. Think for a moment how you devote your life to the Lord. Think of an area of your life that you need to surrender to God. Will you step off the throne and dedicate your life to God?

I believe when we can begin to grasp God's holiness, we will experience a change—personally and corporately. For if we worship God as *Holy, Holy, Holy,* then He would receive complete devotion in all areas of our lives. This transformation and rededication of our lives sounds a lot like revival.

Now as you take your Bible and study God's Word in greater detail, I encourage you to read Job 38-39. Today we looked at how creation can help us grasp the enormity of God. These two chapters in the book of Job contain God's response to Job after he questions God. You will find God asking Job questions, which relate to God's power and authority as Creator of the World. Take time to worship God. Praise Him for His incredible attributes.

Day 2 Health Bite

Today we learned how as believers we choose willingly to worship the Lord. God is God regardless; His worth does not diminish based on our acknowledgement of Him. As believers our goal is to worship God in all aspects of life. This is the spiritual discipline of worship. In the process God transforms and sanctifies us into the persons He desires us to be. *Exercise daily in God—no spiritual flabbiness, please! Workouts in the gymnasium are useful, but a disciplined life in God is far more so, making you fit both today and forever. You can count on this. Take it to heart* (1 Tim. 4:7-8 The Message).

Just like your spiritual health, let your wellness goals infiltrate every area of your life. You probably know of the food-guide pyramid. Today we want you to look at the activity pyramid and pay attention especially to the base level. These are the lifestyle activities. This level is simply doing active things each day beyond the workout. These include yard work, washing the car, taking the stairs, and playing with the kids. The middle sections are the formal workout; the tip of the pyramid is the inactivity level. How much time do you spend watching TV, on the computer, or playing video games? Do these activities sparingly. True wellness is largely determined by the decisions you make about how to live your life.

Challenge: Walk 25 minutes
Do 6 push-ups
Do 20 crunches

Week 3 - Day 3

The Issue of Sin

Memory Verse:

"'Yet a time is coming and has now come when true worshipers will worship the Father in spirit and truth, for they are the kind of worshipers the Father seeks. God is spirit, and his worshipers must worship in spirit and in truth.' The woman said, 'I know that Messiah' (called Christ) 'is coming. When he comes, he will explain everything to us.' Then Jesus declared, 'I who speak to you am he'"
(John 4:23-26).

Today we will concentrate on Isaiah 6:5-7 to study the spiritual discipline of worship. We will focus on this passage: *Then I said, "My destruction is sealed, for I am a sinful man and a member of a sinful race. Yet I have seen the King, the Lord Almighty!"* (Isa. 6:5 The Message).

By confessing sin, Isaiah responds to the glory of the Lord. Today we will see the relationship between sin and worship. The first thing we note from Scripture is that when we are in the presence of God, our sin becomes a blatant problem. Secondly, Isaiah confesses not only his sins but also those of his people. When you understand the holiness of God, confess your sins in response.

What can be done? Along with many other prophets Isaiah tells of a Messiah who would live on earth. Yet, Jesus is not yet here to take away the sins of the world.

Worship leads to forgiveness

Then one of the seraphim flew over to the altar, and he picked up a burning coal with a pair of tongs. He touched my lips with it and said, "See, this coal has touched your lips. Now your guilt is removed, and your sins are forgiven" (Isa. 6:6-7 NLT).

Wow! The enormity of what occurs to Isaiah in that moment often slips past me on initial reading. Almighty God graciously forgives Isaiah's sin and removes his guilt. This gives Isaiah all the more reason to worship the Lord. In the Old Testament people usually sprinkle blood from the sin sacrifices to help restore their relationship with God. However, we see Isaiah receive forgiveness after confessing his sins.

We live in a day in which Isaiah's prophesies are fulfilled through the person of Jesus

Christ. Please turn in your Bible to Romans 10:8-13. Through the study of spiritual disciplines you may have encountered a Holy God. As we see with Isaiah, when we truly understand God's holiness, we cannot help but recognize our sinfulness and shame. Without God's grace and forgiveness we stand condemned. We have not, cannot, and will not accomplish anything that could earn our salvation or erase the impact and consequences of our sin. But Christ—through His life on earth and his death and resurrection—offers a solution to our sin problem (Rom. 6:23). Thus once and for all He pays the price for humanity's sin. Now we face the question of whether to accept God's forgiveness. What about you?

The Bible says in Rom. 10:9-10, *That if you confess with your mouth, "Jesus is Lord," and believe in your heart that God raised him from the dead, you will be saved. For it is with your heart that you believe and are justified, and it is with your mouth that you confess and are saved.* If you have never become a Christian, please do not wait any longer. The practice of spiritual disciplines are a waste of your time otherwise, for they are only works. These help us to grow closer to Christ by learning how to follow Him and helping to establish a lifestyle of commitment. But first you must be saved.

Romans 10:9-10 tells us that after recognizing our sin and need of a Savior we—
1) Confess that Jesus is Lord and believe that God raised Him from the grave.
2) Often people pray a simple prayer to the Lord and state those very things.
3) Now you are saved.

If you just prayed a prayer confessing and believing these things, then you are a child of God. Welcome to the family! I promise you that this is the best choice you ever or will ever make. I am praying for you as you grow in your relationship with God.

Altar of worship

Whether you have followed Christ for many years or just became a Christian, you have received a message of God's grace that changed your life. I mentioned earlier that when we practice the spiritual discipline of worship, we often regularly need to repent of sin. Yet each time we approach the Lord and confess our sin, He forgives us (1 John 1:5-10).

Please open your Bibles and read 1 John 1:5-10.

As you read this passage, what two themes do you see emerge? Describe below.

1)____

____

____

2)____
____
____

The first three verses address the light of God. This light parallels His holiness, just as darkness represents sin. God will shine His light and reveal our dark spots. But the passage also says that when we confess our sin, He will forgive us. Below see how the spiritual discipline of worship helps you mature as you follow Christ.

Practice the Spiritual Discipline of Worship

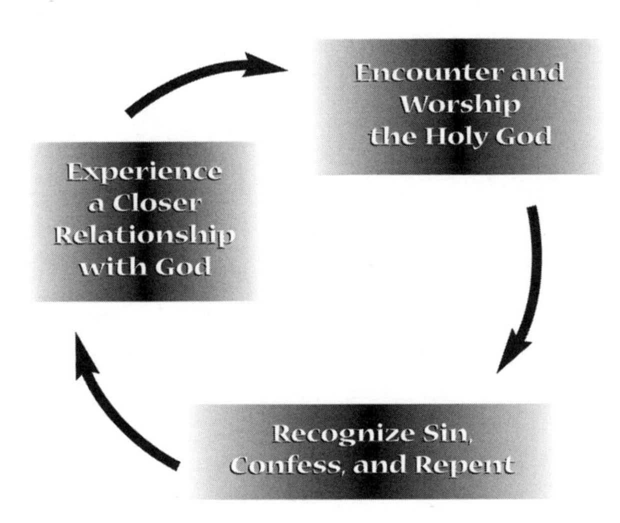

Today as you spend time worshiping God, studying Scripture, and praying, I encourage you to take time to confess sin and praise God for His Holiness, forgiveness, and grace.

Please read 1 Peter 1.

Day 3 Health Bite

Restaurants . . . we are surrounded by businesses that aim to please every palate and lifestyle. Dining out has evolved from a luxury away from the kitchen to an everyday event. We gather, we eat. Dining out is a social experience; if it is done too often, it may lead to an expanding waistline.

Consider these strategies when you eat away from home:
1. Plan ahead. Review the restaurant menu items (nutritional information, if available) online before you arrive; select a healthy option and stick to it when you order. When you order, request a "to-go" container. Before you eat, place part of your meal in it.

2. Focus on portion control, especially with high-fat condiments. The dressing (even the healthy, oil-based kind) on a small side salad can add up to more than 300 calories. Ask for dressings and sauces "on the side" and use sparingly. Use the "Plate Method" (page 46) to ensure a healthy "fuel mix".

3. Practice mindful eating. When we are in a social setting, we may fail to truly "taste" the food or recognize how quickly we eat. Consciously slow down, enjoy every bite, appreciate it, and linger over the meal. Let the pleasure of dining out be about friends or family, not just about the food.

Research confirms that people who eat meals at home are better able to maintain weight.

Choose two to four goals this week to become more mindful of eating "on the go"!

• This week I will limit eating out to ______ times per week.
• I will bring my lunch to work ______ times this week.
• When my meal arrives, I will ask for a to-go container and take ____ (percentage of meal) home in the container.
• I will request dressing and sauces on the side.
Add your own goal here: ____

Week 3 - Day 4

Salvation and Discipleship

Memory Verse:

"'Yet a time is coming and has now come when true worshipers will worship the Father in spirit and truth, for they are the kind of worshipers the Father seeks. God is spirit, and his worshipers must worship in spirit and in truth.' The woman said, 'I know that Messiah' (called Christ) 'is coming. When he comes, he will explain everything to us.' Then Jesus declared, 'I who speak to you am he'"
(John 4:23-26).

In Richard J. Foster's *Streams of Living Water,* he tells the story of young Aurelius, a professor of rhetoric and literature searching for truth, who encountered Ambrose, a Bishop of Milan.

> Ambrose forthrightly declared that Jesus Christ had the power to break the bonds of moral failure. No one had offered that kind of power before . . . Further, Ambrose opened the spiritual meaning of Scripture to Aurelius in a way that released him from a wooden literalism and allowed him to come to the Bible prayerfully, seeking the illumination of the Spirit. Even so, Aurelius was not certain he was quite ready for such soul-shaping commitment. "Give me chastity and self-control," he prayed, "but not yet." All of this was such a mighty struggle for Aurelius because he did not believe, as is so common today, that one could be a convert to Christ without being a disciple of Christ. For him conversion and discipleship were two sides of the same door—and both were necessary to get through the door. In counting the cost, he understood that turning to Christ, meant turning from the intellectual pride that had driven him so fiercely and embracing a lifestyle free of sexual promiscuity. Conversion for Aurelius was no easy assent to a few propositions; it was the restructuring of his whole life. He not only understood that the grace of God was "costly grace"; he was unaware of any other kind of grace. . . . I am telling you the story of Aurelius Augustine, later to become the famous bishop of Hippo."[1]

How do we respond to the gospel? If we accept it, do we continue living the same way? Or do we change?

Today, in Isaiah 6:8-13, we continue our study of worship. We will specifically look at how salvation affects a life. Please read this passage.

Who will go?

In verse 8 we first see a question about who will serve the Lord. Isaiah eagerly responds to the call. The spiritual discipline of service will be our study topic next week. Yet here in Isaiah 6 we find the link between these two disciplines.

At this point Isaiah does not know his future job assignment nor the response of the people. He merely has an encounter with the Almighty God and receives forgiveness. He volunteers to tell others about the truth he knows and experiences.

The call to tell the truth about the gospel and the salvation Christ brought is one that all Christians have. Think back to the time when you became a Christian. Did you find that sharing about Christ was easy?

For what type of service did I volunteer?

So why does God have to ask? After studying this passage and various commentaries, I found that many theologians agreed that God had chosen Isaiah as His servant—a servant who would speak a message from the Lord.

But God still asks. All Christ followers have the opportunity to respond with a life of service. God selects us, but we agree to volunteer for service.

"*Whom shall I send? And who will go for us?*" says Isaiah 6:8b NIV. Here we find an Old Testament use of *God* in the plural. This shows the involvement of the Trinity: the Father, Son, and Holy Spirit.[2]

Last week I told you about how God convicted me about forgiveness. I mentioned that as His child—a new creation, completely forgiven for my un-payable debt—I am expected to respond toward others with forgiveness. Yet for a while I struggled to trust the church, especially with my family. By accepting a call to the ministry I believed it would open my family up for mistreatment.

After about a decade, God tugged on my heart and asked again, "*Who should I send?*" I finally responded, as Isaiah did, "*Here I am; send me*."

Like Isaiah, God may call you to a task; afterward you will find what that task entails. Some of you may know ahead of time what are some of the risks to obeying Christ in a specific way.

Around the world many people face emotional, physical, and/or financial costs for believing in and following Christ (Luke 14:25-35). My experience of persecution would appear laughable to them.

When we encounter the Holy God and His amazing grace, why do we hesitate to give Him our all? Like Augustine, I don't know of any other kind of grace.

When we encounter a Holy God whose power fills the entire earth, our strength and the risks seem to diminish in size. God can use the spiritual discipline of worship as a time to soften our hearts and prepare us to go out and work. By serving, sharing about Christ, and discipling others, we can bring glory to the God we love to worship.

Meditate on the words to the familiar hymn, *When I Survey the Wondrous Cross:*

When I survey the wondrous cross,
On which the Prince of glory died,
My richest gain I count but loss,
And pour contempt on all my pride.

Forbid it, Lord, that I should boast,
Save in the death of Christ my God;
All the vain things that charm me most,
I sacrifice them to his blood.

See, from his head, his hands, his feet,
Sorrow and love flow mingled down;
Did e'er such love and sorrow meet,
Or thorns compose so rich a crown.

Were the whole realm of nature mine,
That were a present far too small;
Love so amazing, so divine,
Demands my soul, my life, my all.[3]

AMEN.

(Gal. 6:14. Words, Isaac Watts, 1707. Tune HAMBURG, Lowell Mason, 1824)

Please read John 21. Here we find the resurrected Jesus meeting with His disciples.

Day 4 Health Bite

The spiritual discipline of worshiping God on your own helps prepare your heart for corporate worship. In exercise, you make personal preparation to help ready yourself for a game or a workout. To begin with, you need a few essentials—shoes, shirt, and shorts. Make sure your clothes are comfortable and somewhat loose. Special shoes are necessary. Worn-out basketball or old tennis shoes may cause injury. Walking or running shoes have a specially designed heel for absorbing shock. The shoe should have a firm arch-support, a flexible sole, and extra room for your toes. To obtain a good fit, acquire these at a reputable sporting-goods store. A good pair should last about 500-600 miles.

In all things remember your goal: *Strip down, start running—and never quit! Keep your eyes on Jesus, who both began and finished this race we're in* (Heb. 12:1-2). Don't forget that the most difficult part of working out is putting on your shoes!

Challenge: Take the 1-mile walk test.
Do 6 push-ups.
Do 20 crunches.

Week 3 - Day 5

True Worshipers

Memory Verse:

"'Yet a time is coming and has now come when true worshipers will worship the Father in spirit and truth, for they are the kind of worshipers the Father seeks. God is spirit, and his worshipers must worship in spirit and in truth.' The woman said, 'I know that Messiah' (called Christ) 'is coming. When he comes, he will explain everything to us.' Then Jesus declared, 'I who speak to you am he'"
(John 4:23-26).

This week we looked at Isaiah's encounter with the Holy God to study the spiritual discipline of worship. Isaiah operates under the sacrificial system of the old covenant. When Christ is on earth, He brings a new covenant and with it a new way of worship.

Please turn to John 4 in your Bible. We will focus on verses 21-26, but for contextual purposes read John 4:1-26 and answer the following questions.

In this scenario, where was Jesus?

____

What time of day did Jesus sit down at the well?

____

With whom did Jesus strike up a conversation?

____

Why was she shocked when Jesus spoke to her?

____

For what did Jesus ask her?

____

What type of water did Jesus tell her He had?

____

Why do you think this woman went to draw water in the heat of the day?

____

____

What did Jesus tell her about her past?

How did the Samaritan woman avoid an awkward conversation?

After you answer these questions, you have now reached our primary passage for today. As you look at the context, you may think this woman chases a theological rabbit-trail just to avoid a personal topic—her history with men. But Jesus uses her question to teach us about worship and to explain the new covenant He brought.

Location

The Samaritan woman wants to know where to worship. Second Kings 17:24-41 tells the story of the Samaritan beginnings. Sargon of Assyria invades Israel; he takes many Jewish exiles and brings captives from other lands to live with the few remaining Israelites. These replaced captives do not worship the God of the Israelites. Second Kings tell us that the Lord sends out a lion to kill some of them because of their pagan worship. Therefore they begin to follow Jewish religious customs while they maintain their pagan practices. The Israelites living in the land marry the foreign captives; the Samaritans are their descendants.

The Samaritan woman may have believed that if she just worshiped where God commanded, then He would be appeased. Her belief may have originated from the attitude of her culture—a desire to adapt but not change their worship to a point in which they worship only the one true God.

Do you see this mindset in our world today? If so, describe how.

Our Western culture does not lack for religiosity. Yet I find we hold a striking resemblance to the Samaritans. Our choices may result from a desire to appease and not from one of complete surrender.

Have you found that "non-Christian beliefs" may wear sheep's clothing and seem to bear very little difference from "Christian beliefs"? What examples of this do you see in your life?

Thankfully Jesus takes the Samaritan woman's conversational detour as a chance to teach about true worship. Please re-read John 4:21-26. He does not answer her question on location but rather describes for Jews, Samaritans, and all others, including us, what characterizes a true worshiper.

Worship is not about location. Jesus clearly states in John 4:21-23 that the time has arrived for a new kind of worship—one based on spirit and truth instead of place.

Spirit

When you hear the term *spirit*, how would you describe it? Many times our thoughts link the word *spirit* or *spiritual* to our culture's definition—one of meditation or emptying your spirit of negative thoughts or energy.

Scripture speaks of the spirit in a different way. Yesterday, we saw briefly a reference to the Trinity: the one, true, Holy God consisting of the Father, the Son, and the Holy Spirit (Isa. 6:8). As Christians, Jesus tells us that He will go and send a Counselor, the Spirit, that guides us in all truth. He does this (John 14:15-31 and Acts 2:32-33).

This Spirit lives within us, directs us, and teaches us. The Holy Spirit indwells all believers; this is how Christ intended for us to worship during the time of the new covenant—we worship in the spirit.

We can worship many things. But true worshipers must have the Holy Spirit. This introduces Jesus' qualification of truth. For after we have faith in Christ, we receive the Holy Spirit. The Spirit helps us to discern truth. Christ is the central focus of that truth.

Truth

In today's information age we struggle to know the truth. With a never-ending list of possible sources, how do we sort the information and factor what is truth? In John 4, Jesus explains the kind of worshipers God wants. The Samaritan woman still responds with uncertainty. She knows of a promised Messiah Who will provide truth (John 4:25).

Here we have a specific instance where Jesus clearly claims to be the Messiah. He states blatantly, "I who speak to you am he" (John 4:26).

We see in these two verses how truth must emanate from the Messiah and that Jesus is the Christ. Therefore, our source of truth in life and in worship must be based on Jesus Christ. The best resource for us, therefore, is the Bible and specifically the gospels to explain to us truth.

John 4:23-24 says, *Yet a time is coming and has now come when the true worshipers will worship the Father in spirit and truth, for they are the kind of worshipers the Father seeks.*

A Christ-follower practicing the spiritual discipline of worship must believe in Scripture's teaching about truth—Christ—and live by the direction of the Holy Spirit. Then our worship, whether in a church service or Monday morning at the office, will be pleasing to the Father.

Revelation 4 and 5 provide us with a view into heaven in which God sits enthroned. We can observe the heavenly worship service of the one, true God. Today please take some time to read these chapters and to reflect on the awesome God you serve.

Day 5 Health Bite

Congratulations. You are achieving great progress through your journey toward making health and wellness a greater priority! Let's take this time to celebrate your success, identify obstacles, and revisit the motivation that is propelling you to continue on.

As we previously discussed, goal-setting is essential to keep you on track to meet your vision for a healthier life. Take a moment to look back on the goals you set during the last two weeks. What percent of the time were you able to meet your goals? If you were unable to meet them 75 percent of the time, determine what obstacles or "roadblocks" prevented you from achieving the goal. Do not feel guilty; use this as a learning opportunity to evaluate how you can do things differently in the upcoming week.

If you met the goals greater than 75 percent, celebrate! Then consider whether this is a goal you can continue to do and eventually make a life habit! I challenge you as you move into week four to re-evaluate what motivates you to continue healthy habits.

Goals: **(List your prior goals, with the percentage complete)**

Week 1: (percentage complete) Identify obstacles or successes!

____

____

Week 2: (percentage complete)

____

____

Week 3: (percentage complete)

____

____

After you evaluate your progress, look forward. Think about what you have learned during the past three weeks and set two to four new goals (or re-establish old goals) toward which you would like to work.

GOAL 1:

GOAL 2:

GOAL 3:

GOAL 4:

Week 4 - Day 1

Our Savior Serves

Memory Verse:

"You call me 'Teacher' and "Lord," and rightly so, for that is what I am. Now that I, your Lord and Teacher, have washed your feet, you also should wash one another's feet. I have set for you an example that you should do as I have done for you. I tell you the truth, no servant is greater than his master, nor is a messenger greater than the one who sent him. Now that you know these things, you will be blessed if you do them" (John 13:13-17).

We begin our study of the spiritual discipline of service from a very common passage—John 13, in which Jesus washes the disciples' feet.

Please take the time to read John 13:1-17.

Christ's purpose

Jesus knew He was sent to earth to die. *His hour had come that He should depart out of this world to the Father, having loved His own who were in the world, He loved them to the end* (John 13:1b NASB). In John 13 Jesus sets an example of service for us to follow. Here we find Him focused on His goal. Jesus' life does not compare to the rest of humanity because He was fully God and fully human. However, we can approach service with the same goal-centered intention. As believers we know our basic purpose in life—to know our Savior and live in obedience to Him (John 3:16-17 and Matt. 16:24).

Part of our obedience involves the discipline of service (John 13:13-17).

When you approach service, how is your attitude? What are your motives? Why do you do it?

____

____

____

Christ's love

In John 13:1, we next see Christ's love. Think about God's undeserved and unwavering love for His children.

John 13:2 tells of a subplot to Jesus' example of service. What has occurred before the evening meal? What significance does this play?

___

___

___

The disciples likely expect a memorable Passover meal with their Teacher and Lord. But none of the disciples truly understand the events that will occur that day. Even Judas Iscariot does not realize the significance of his betrayal. A spiritual war already rages.

Do you think your acts of service have more importance than does the surface-level, meeting of a need? If so, why?

___

___

___

Our acts of service could never compare with those of Christ. However, many times we face a decision of whether to love in an evil world. What will you choose?

Please read Romans 12:17-21. In this passage, what does Paul tell us to do?

___

___

___

Intentional humility

John 13:3 exposes the truth that Jesus knows He is God Almighty, the Redeemer/Messiah sent to save the world. Scripture tells us that Jesus Christ has authority over all things!

Jesus knows His purpose; He knows about the spiritual warfare; He knows He possesses all authority. So what does He do next? He serves. *So he got up from the meal, took off his outer clothing, and wrapped a towel around his waist. After that, he poured water into a basin and began to wash his disciples' feet, drying them with the towel that was wrapped around him (*John 13:4-5).

Not only does Jesus serve, He takes the most undesirable role—foot-washing. He does the job of Gentile slaves—the job even Jewish slaves pass off to others. He humbles Himself.

Serving with humility

Last week we looked at the spiritual discipline of worship. Worshiping God should automatically stir in us a realization of who we are and what a helpless state we are in without the mercy and grace of God.

How do we transfer a humble attitude formed in worship to the discipline of service?

____

____

Basically we recognize reality. *But whoever lives by the truth comes into the light, so that it may be seen plainly that what he has done has been done through God* (John 3:21).

Here we find this matter explained. We can serve with humility and live accomplishing good with the help of God. Even our acts of service give credit to our Savior.

After the Lord's Supper, Jesus and the disciples leave for the olive grove to pray. Judas arrives later with officers and religious leaders to arrest Him. By the end of the evening His disciples desert Him; one disowns Him three times. Jesus knows this beforehand yet loves them anyway.

Take a moment to reflect on Jesus' love and sacrifice. Briefly write down a prayer of thanksgiving for His love and service (Rom. 5:18-21 and 2 Cor. 5:13-15).

____

____

____

____

____

Serving today

Christ serves as our perfect example. Today He continues to use people to show His love to others.

Think about the people who show God's love to you. List one person who can serve as a role model for you.

____

Now make a list of ways that you can serve in your church and sphere of influence. Specifically think of a challenging situation to which you can respond with love instead of evil.

____
____
____
____

Each one should use whatever gift he has received to serve others, faithfully administering God's grace in its various forms (1 Pet. 4:10).

Tabitha, otherwise known as Dorcas, a disciple of Christ in Joppa, lived serving others. In the New Testament she passes away; God uses Peter to raise her from the dead.

Please read her story in Acts 9:36-43 about how the influence of her love and service influenced her community.

Day 1 Health Bite

Experts have estimated that 21 days are required to form a habit. So how are you doing? Do you have more energy, feel more "comfortable in your own skin", or have confidence that you are taking a pro-active approach to improve your health? If the answer is *YES,* then share your success with friends, family, or strangers!

A dear Christian friend calls me monthly to ask if I would like to "break bread" with him! I like his term *breaking bread.* It transcends me back into the New Testament, as I envision Jesus relaxing and eating with the disciples. Sharing a home-cooked meal with friends or family can be a special event and an act of service.

Would you be willing to share your favorite recipe (or even try a new one) this week?

These may help you discover a new delicious creation:
www.cookinglight.com
www.eatingwell.com
www.allrecipes.com
www.americanheartassociation.org

How could you use food to serve?

Consider these suggestions:
1. Invite friends or family for dinner. Share one positive change you have made that has impacted your health!
2. Take a meal to a person who is homebound, financially struggling, or in need of company.
3. Volunteer to take a snack or dessert to your Bible study. Be creative! Take food that would benefit the health of all who attend.
4. Get involved in an outreach group that feeds the homeless.
5. "Break bread" with your role model who exemplifies Christian service. Discuss how his or her service has impacted your life.

What is your plan for this week?

____

____

____

____

Week 4 - Day 2

Reversing Roles

Memory Verse:

"You call me 'Teacher' and 'Lord,' and rightly so, for that is what I am. Now that I, your Lord and Teacher, have washed your feet, you also should wash one another's feet. I have set for you an example that you should do as I have done for you. I tell you the truth, no servant is greater than his master, nor is a messenger greater than the one who sent him. Now that you know these things, you will be blessed if you do them" (John 13:13-17).

Please turn in your Bible to John 13:6-8 and read this passage.

Peter struggled to understand the message of Jesus' teaching. Peter followed the tradition at that time of honoring teachers and rabbis. He did not envision his Teacher humbling Himself in such a way. The role reversal seemed too dramatic.

I believe that we, as people in a Western culture, still struggle with a role reversal similar to that of Peter—except that we may have expectations of the treatment we should receive or the jobs we want to do.

Let's evaluate ourselves. Below I have listed seven questions. Fill them out to evaluate how well you practice the spiritual discipline of service. Ahead of time, decide not to use this activity to fuel your pride.

1. On a 1-to-10 scale, with 1 being poor and 10 being excellent, how do you rank yourself as willingness to serve when an opportunity arrives? ______

2. Describe your last act of service toward a loved one.

____

____

3. Think about the last time someone requested a favor or act of service that you believed took too much of your time or energy or a time your ego cringed when the person asked you to do it. What happened?

____

____

____

4. Do you have a household task that you consider beneath you?

____

____

5. What about professionally? Do you consider yourself superior to co-workers or friends whose vocational roles differ from yours?

____

____

____

6. What about at church? Do you find yourself favoring some individuals and ignoring others?

____

A good listener has a better chance at service. Before you launch into a project, listen to those you serve. Recognize a real need; seek a way to meet the need. An active listener is one who hears the speaker and then bases his or her actions on the speaker's message

7. On a scale of 1 to 10, with 1 being poor and 10 excellent, how would you rank yourself as an active listener? ___

Personal evaluation

Many people do not know of Jesus Christ. God uses the church as His vessel in the world. Thankfully, today God has His people around the world shining the light of the gospel and living a message of love. Remember: you play an important role in God's work!

Yet, I struggle with three terrible characteristics: pride, selfishness, and apathy. In a world often unfamiliar with the teaching of Jesus, I find that others look to us—His followers—as an example. Service can represent God's love and teaching to others. Regular evaluation of my goals and success in acting on them helps me to live intentionally.

I pray that in my life and yours God would soften our hearts and give us a passion to love and serve others. Let us get moving and serve more tomorrow than we did today!

Please read James 2. This passage tells how to relate to those within the church and addresses acts of service in the world. Think about what both lessons teach about attitude and actions.

Day 2 Health Bite

Service impacts all areas of your life, but it especially impacts close family and friends. The small acts of service that often go unnoticed help to build up your family, and on a more broad arena, the church.

Today we want you to think of service as you would walking. It has a cumulative effect. Walking is a fitness activity that requires moderate effort. Over a period of time these daily walks make significant contribution to our general health and overall fitness. We can use a small device called a *pedometer* to measure the distance of these bouts of work. Much as our service to others does, over time the long-term daily input accumulates. Just as the pedometer logs in the miles, our desire to serve builds up the body of Christ. The New American Standard Bible in Galatians 5:13 says, *But through love, serve one another.*

A pedometer is a popular device people use to track their physical activity patterns. It provides information about the number of steps a person takes. Stride length and weight can be entered into most pedometers to provide estimates of distance traveled and/or calories burned. About 10,000 steps (5 miles) has been promoted as the standard for activity level, but this distance may be too difficult for some and not tough enough for others.

Start by finding your baseline—how many steps you take in a normal day. Then add 10 percent each week until you reach your goal.

Another device that you might find helpful is a heart-rate monitor. A watch (receiver), usually worn on the wrist, receives a signal from a transmitter attached to a strap worn around the chest. The monitor displays heart rate and allows the exerciser to maintain his or her target rate.

Challenge: Walk 35 minutes.
Do 8 push-ups.
Do 25 crunches.

Week 4 - Day 3

A Servant's Mentality

Memory Verse:

"You call me 'Teacher' and "Lord," and rightly so, for that is what I am. Now that I, your Lord and Teacher, have washed your feet, you also should wash one another's feet. I have set for you an example that you should do as I have done for you. I tell you the truth, no servant is greater than his master, nor is a messenger greater than the one who sent him. Now that you know these things, you will be blessed if you do them" (John 13:13-17).

For today's look at the spiritual discipline of service, please read Luke 17:7-10.

In these three verses we find a mentality about service that we rarely see in our Western culture. Yet, here we find a teaching from Jesus. As His followers we can use this as a reality check.

Deserve versus duty

In this short passage Jesus first gives the setting: a servant who works in the fields tending to the crops and sheep.

Jesus then asks three questions. Below please list the questions He asks.

1)____
____

2) ____
____

3) ____
____

This passage cuts at the heart of an issue about service. Why do we do it? Do we serve out of duty or to get a reward?

Think for a moment of the motivation for you. Do you ever believe that because you served, you deserve a specific recognition or reward?

____

What if the reward or recognition never arrives? How do you respond?

____

____

Do you ever find yourself waiting for the moment in which you will receive the special treatment? This passage does not state that giving encouragement and thanks for service is wrong. But it cuts to the heart of our view of service. It reveals our motives. The Bible says, *The Lord's searchlight penetrates the human spirit, exposing every hidden motive* (Prov. 20:27 NLT).

Today please spend some time in study, prayer, and meditation. I pray that during this time, the Lord will help to reveal your motives. You then can repent of them and surrender your service to the Lord.

A dutiful servant serves faithfully in all circumstances. Please read Matthew 25:31-46.

This week serve the Lord in a way in which you know no one will pay you back—an unrecognized and unrewarded act. Take time to evaluate Matthew 25 and Luke 17 and your real-life experience.

Day 3 Health Bite

Food labels—helpful or hazardous to your sanity? That small print on the side of your favorite snack food can be confusing! The prior lesson discussed how to balance "whole" foods, but what about "pre-packaged" food? Intentionally learn to translate the food label for the purpose of achieving your health and wellness goals! Become a savvy food label reader.

SERVING SIZE: The label information relates to the serving size, not the entire package.

FAT: Limit saturated fat and trans fat that can lead to chronic disease.
• Limit 2 grams of saturated fat per serving
• Select food with 0 trans fat; avoid products that list "partially hydrogenated oil" in the first five ingredients.
• Ultimate goal: less than 10-15 grams saturated; less than than 1 gram trans-fat

SODIUM: Canned items and packet seasonings are notorious for salt. These lead to high blood pressure and fluid retention.
• Look for less than 300 mg or less per serving (less than 250 mg if you have hypertension)
• Pre-packaged meals: less than 650 mg sodium
• Ultimate goal: less than 3,000 mg sodium per day (less than 2,000 if you have hypertension)

FIBER: Most Americans fall short on fiber!
• Choose whole grains with more than 3 grams
• Choose cereals with more than 5 grams
• Eat a plant-based diet rich with at least six servings of fruits and veggies.
• Ultimate goal: 25-35 grams per day

SUGAR: Attempt to limit foods with "added" sugars.
• Limit 10 grams sugar in most foods (except milk and yogurt that contain "natural" milk sugar— keep these less than 20 grams per serving)
• If sugar, high-fructose syrup, or corn syrup is in first five ingredients, use sparingly
• Ultimate goal: less than 10 teaspoons per day of "added sugar" (1 teaspoon of sugar = 4 grams, so this would mean limiting to 40 grams)

Percentage Daily Value: If the nutrient listed is over 10 percent, that means it is a significant source of that nutrient.

Use these strategies at least 85 percent of the time. You will be on your way to selecting healthier pre-packaged food!

Week 4 - Day 4

Spiritual Gifts

Memory Verse:

"You call me 'Teacher' and 'Lord,' and rightly so, for that is what I am. Now that I, your Lord and Teacher, have washed your feet, you also should wash one another's feet. I have set for you an example that you should do as I have done for you. I tell you the truth, no servant is greater than his master, nor is a messenger greater than the one who sent him. Now that you know these things, you will be blessed if you do them" (John 13:13-17).

When we discuss service in the church, talking about spiritual gifts becomes imperative. As believers we make up the body of Christ (Rom. 12:4). In 1 Corinthians 12, Paul writes about spiritual gifts given to each member. He clarifies their source and purpose.

Spiritual source

Paul writes 1 Corinthians to provide church discipline. He addresses the church because it acts selfishly and divisively. This originates from two places: 1) selfish pride and 2) false teaching. To correct the people's dysfunction, Paul teaches them about the "spirituality" of the spiritual gifts.

Please take a moment and read 1 Corinthians 12:1-3. What do you see as the qualifier for whether someone's teaching lines up with the Spirit of God?

____

____

____

The source of the spiritual gifts must be God. But to determine whether a gift or the person claiming a gift is legitimate or false, find out what he or she says about Jesus, the second part of the Trinity. Does the individual call Him *Lord*: fully God and fully human? If not, then dismiss the person as a false teacher.

Do you find other spiritual sources in our world today that at first appear acceptable? What do they claim about Christ?

____

____

____

Now take a moment to read 1 Corinthians 12:4-6. Based on this verse fill out the spaces in the chart below.

Different kinds of . . .	But the same . . .

In these three verses we see two things: 1) The unity of the Trinity working with the church, and 2) The variety of ministries available.

This passage tells us that the Holy Spirit, the Son—Jesus Christ—and God the Father all three play an active, unified role in the church. They all work together through the giving, manifestation, and work of the church through spiritual gifts.

Manifestation of the Spirit (1 Cor. 12:7-11)

Paul tells us that spiritual gifts originate from the same God, but they may show themselves in different ways. Take a moment and list the spiritual gifts Paul mentions in 1 Corinthians 12:7-10. This is not an exhaustive list (Eph. 4:11 and Rom. 12:3-8).

____

____

____

Do you know which spiritual gift(s) the Lord gave you? If so, please write it (them) here.

____

____

In the space provided please write 1 Corinthians 12:7. Circle the reason the Holy Spirit gives us spiritual gifts.

____

____

Natural versus spiritual

Think for a moment about one of your natural talents. Below write it down.

____

For a while I struggled to know whether natural talents were the same or different from spiritual gifts. In 1 Corinthians 12 we find that a spiritual gift is given after one acknowledges Jesus Christ as his or her Lord (1 Cor. 12:3).

In the Old Testament we see several figures who serve the Lord and are described as receiving a natural talent from the Spirit of God. Bezalel and Oholiab are two examples; they serve as master craftsmen assigned to the task of building the tabernacle (Ex. 31-39).

On the other hand, Cyrus, king of Persia, excels as leader and administrator. He sends the exiled Jews back to Jerusalem to build the temple. We do not know of his faith in God. Yet, we cannot question his unique place in God's plan (2 Chron. 36:22-23).

Instances such as this lead me to believe that natural talents are from God because He created us; yet one does not have to claim Christ as Lord in order to have them.

The common link lies in their source. God gave us both talents and spiritual gifts. He deserves praise for both.

The "walkalator"

All these are the work of one and the same Spirit, and he gives them to each one, just as he determines (1 Cor. 12:11).

My dad once compared spiritual gifts to a moving sidewalk at an airport, otherwise known as a *walkalator*. If you went walking down a long corridor in an airport, you may find a walkway in the middle with a walkalator on either side; it moves in opposite directions. Typically if people need to accomplish a task, such as making their flight on time, they will take the walkalator while they maintain their previous walking pace. If you were to watch them, they cover significantly more ground than if they just kept up their pace on the middle pathway.

In the same way, spiritual gifts help us to accomplish more than if we were to complete a task in our own strength. Yet if someone were to look at your life, that person wouldn't recognize the walker but rather that the Holy Spirit is enabling the individual to serve in a specific capacity to build up the church.

Today read Romans 12:1-8 to learn more about spiritual gifts. Think about ways you could serve to build up the church. Make plans to use your spiritual gift(s) this month. Below write the plan.

____

____

Day 4 Health Bite

Let's talk about the role of your heart, the organ that literally sustains life. After a courageous performance in sports, people often say, "He's got heart!" This is the supreme compliment to a performer because of the importance of the heart to the entire body.

The heart is the life-sustaining pump that begins to beat before birth and continues until your last breath. It must be strong; you must care for it. The spiritual journey is more than salvation. Accepting Christ as our Savior is our spiritual birth. Then we must work daily to serve the Lord and do his will. This is a journey of endurance. Hebrews 10:36 says, *For you need endurance in order to do God's will* (NET Bible).

To get the most out of your workout, you will need to find your target heart rate. After a short warmup, the heart rate should be elevated and maintained into the target zone for a specified period of time. It will be short in the beginning and gradually extend to 30-45 minutes.

Using the chart on page 187, determine your target heart-rate zone.

Challenge: Walk for 40 minutes.
Do 8 push-ups.
Do 40 crunches.

Week 4 - Day 5

Many Members

Memory Verse:

"You call me 'Teacher' and 'Lord,' and rightly so, for that is what I am. Now that I, your Lord and Teacher, have washed your feet, you also should wash one another's feet. I have set for you an example that you should do as I have done for you. I tell you the truth, no servant is greater than his master, nor is a messenger greater than the one who sent him. Now that you know these things, you will be blessed if you do them" (John 13:13-17).

Please open your Bible to 1 Corinthians 12:14-19. What situation do you see Paul addressing?

____

____

Here we find that members of the church placed guidelines on how they would serve and on when they would serve.

Yesterday we learned that spiritual gifts are from God as He decides (1 Cor. 12:11). Again in 1 Corinthians 12:18 Paul reminds us of this. So what happens? Likely, the church members forget the source of their gifts.

To investigate this concept further please turn to and read Matthew 25:14-30. From this parable we learn three things about the kingdom of God. Below fill in the blanks.

1) The M__________ distributes the talents (Matt. 25:14-15).
2) He does not distribute the talents in e__________ quantity (Matt. 25:15).
3) Regardless of the servants' use of the t___________, the servants all are responsible for their actions (Matt. 25:19-30).

Based on Matthew 25, how far would the believers' selfish plan get them? *But in fact God has arranged the parts in the body, every one of them, just as he wanted them to be* (1 Cor. 12:18).

Interdependence

Please read 1 Corinthians 12:21-26.

These verses describe how the church should seek equality of respect for each part. It describes how we encourage each other's strengths and support each other in our weaknesses.

Think about a church group with whom you have ministered. How did you see this mentality of encouragement and support acted out when you served together?

____

____

____

1 Cor. 12:25 says *so there should be no division in the body, but that its parts should have equal concern for each other.*

Do you see any divisiveness in the church that you attend? If so, what could you do to show equal concern for each other?

____

____

If you do not see divisiveness—excellent! Work for unity by caring for everyone equally.

A part

*Now you are the body of Christ, and each one of you is part of it (*1 Cor. 12:27).
In this verse we find the use of the plural *you.* We exist as a part, a member of the body of Christ.

In our Western world, many of us live independently and often view ourselves in the same manner. Yet this mentality does not transfer well to the church. Instead of being fancy-free, this mentality reveals self-centeredness. Paul writes in response to false teaching within the church. The false teachers serve and speak to benefit themselves. Their first problem is that they don't view Christ as Lord. Thus secondly, they do not live and serve as He intends. They do not consider the parts working together in unity.

The Corinthian church lived in a society known for intellectual wisdom and one that is religiously pluralistic, with rampant immorality. Do you recognize these characteristics in our world today? 1 Corinthians 12:27 reminds us not to transition this or a similar mentality to the use of spiritual gifts in the church. Instead, it tells us that the body, designed by God, is meant to relate in an interdependent manner.

Fit to serve

This Bible study had its origin after I heard a sermon series on church wellness. I mentioned to my church that since I majored in nutrition, I had given nutrition presentations at a couple of churches. The church let me teach a four-week class. The first time I taught it, Don and Carol Mathus, our exercise writers, attended the class.

Later that spring God brought the opportunity of putting this Bible study into a book. I started praying about what it should include, because we hoped to expand the course. Very soon God revealed to me that I needed to include the help of other health experts who were followers of Christ. So I called the Mathuses and Julie Bender, our nutrition writer. Before long we began writing this book. All the various contributors to this study work together as a whole.

What about you?

In writing this study, we hope you will see that the church needs all of its parts to work together. We represent only four parts of the body of Christ. Think about what role you play in serving the Lord. God has a plan to use all of His children.

Please read 1 Corinthians 12:28-31. Paul begins with, *And in the church God has appointed* . . . (1 Cor. 12:28a). We find Paul repeats for the third time that God determines our gifting.[1] In conclusion, God gives us spiritual gifts so that we can serve as unique and interdependent members of the body of Christ. An active member leads to a healthy body. Is the body fit to serve?

John 13 told of Christ's example and taught us about service. 1 Corinthians 12 describes the source and purpose of spiritual gifts use for ministering or serving the church. 1 Corinthians 13, the famous love chapter, follows immediately behind a lesson on the spiritual gifts—in part, to tell that emphasis is not placed on the gifts but on our new way of life as followers of Christ.

Please read 1 Corinthians 13 and meditate on the relationship between love and spiritual discipline of service. Because the order of these two passages shows us the importance of linking love with service, please consider reading Romans 12:1-21, too.

Day 5 Health Bite

Focusing on our strengths can be a source of great encouragement to continue our healthy habits; unfortunately we tend to dwell on our failures. Take time to write down some of your healthy habits of which you are proud.

Take inventory—focus on the good! Write a note of thanks to the Lord, Who helped you to adopt these healthy habits. Keep in mind: small changes can lead to significant, long-term differences in your health and in your risk of disease.

Health habits I am proud that I do consistently:

____

____

____

____

Goals I have been working on throughout the past four weeks and that I have been able to do consistently:

____

____

____

____

This weekend celebrate your success!

Week 5 - Day 1

Waiting on an Involuntary Muscle

Memory Verse:

"Then Haggai, the Lord's messenger, gave this message of the Lord to the people: 'I am with you,' declares the Lord" (Hag. 1:13).

May of my senior year in high school finally arrived. I left school on a Monday with my final-exam exemptions in hand. The parties were planned; my cap and gown sat waiting at home. I had prepared myself to sit back and enjoy the last couple of weeks with all their festivities and ceremonies.

After dinner I started feeling sick. Before long I knew something was wrong. My older brother and a neighbor took me to the emergency room. Mom and Dad had attended church activities that evening, so they just met us at the hospital.

At first, the doctors weren't quite sure what went wrong, so they transferred me to a children's hospital. The doctors discovered that the scar tissue from the diaphragmatic hernia surgery I had at birth completely blocked part of my small intestine. I needed surgery immediately.

In the morning after surgery, the doctors stopped by to tell us the typical recovery time and encouraged me that a few days are usually necessary for intestines to wake back up. Then I could go home. I took this as great news, since previously, when sick, if I followed all of the doctor's orders, I usually got to go home faster than predicted. This remained my plan, since all of our senior-class festivities would occur within the next two weeks. I did not want to miss them.

The days slowly passed. The medical personal could give me nothing to wake my intestines. They had no magic little pill. They advised me to walk around the hospital floor and wait. So I walked and waited. Each day the doctors would stop by and listen to my intestines for any noise. But my intestines were silent.

Two weeks post-op, I remained in the same place with the same prognosis. I asked the doctors to unplug the IV's and let me at least go to the graduation ceremony. They told me that to do so would interfere with my progress. So we agreed to forgo graduation. College orientation—two days away—became my next goal

.

The night before orientation I remained in the hospital. My mom and I prayed and read the Bible together. Then she turned off the lights and slept in the hospital recliner.

I did not sleep. Instead, I took this as a moment to seek God . . . alone. Habitually during the last week I had lain awake to read or pray and search for a Word from God. *Why would now be different?* I wondered. Each night I tuned my ears to hear from Him, but He remained silent, just like my intestines had.

So in the glow of the IV pumps I pulled out my Bible. If I held it up just right, I had enough light. After perusing the Old Testament, I stopped at Lamentations. *This fits,* I thought. So I read about Jeremiah and his five dirges—the funeral songs, as Babylon attacked Jerusalem and killed and destroyed the people.

Lamentations 3 struck a chord with me. This was Jeremiah's personal dirge—his own cry to God.

The next morning arrived quickly; the doctors were there bright and early for rounds. They thought they heard gurgling. So they quickly rushed me to radiology; my intestines looked as though they were waking up. Within an hour the doctors told me that I could leave the hospital as long as I tolerated some food. For 16 days I had not eaten anything. The medical personnel fed me through an IV in my arm, since nourishment needed to avoid my intestines. Eating and tolerating the meal was the only thing between college orientation and me. Fortunately that morning I was able to take food by mouth and tolerate it satisfactorily.

In no time my parents and brother loaded me in the car; we drove down to Waco for the Baylor orientation. We got there just in time for the opening meeting. My cousin, Julie, one of my best friends, just happened to have orientation at the same time, so we stayed near each other in case I got a little woozy. That evening Julie and I met up with our families. We headed back to the hotel to rest.

Hope

Please open up your Bible and read Lamentations 3.

During a time of suffering, Jeremiah seeks God in solitude. He recalls that his faithful God is his only source of salvation. In a moment of solitude I, too, remembered that my only hope is from God.

Lamentations 3:19-33 specifically hit home. These verses illustrated the process I went through that night in the hospital room. God's Word guided me through my time of solitude. God whispered a Word of hope to my heart.

Take a moment and write down what these verses show about the transition in Jeremiah's attitude.

____

____

____

____

An easy solution for unplanned events

Frequently I meet stress eaters; in fact, I, myself, notice a tendency to let my circumstances impact my eating habits. However, by making an intentional practice of the spiritual discipline of solitude, you may find yourself planning to seek the Lord instead of food. We can use many things to debrief from the challenges of life. Sometimes food presents an easy escape, because we can seek to suppress the challenges alone without anyone's help.

Lamentations showed me I could acknowledge reality and grieve; I did not have to do this in front of a watching world. When we practice the spiritual discipline of solitude, we are not alone, because we run to the feet of our Savior.

Jeremiah grieved, but he spoke a word of hope. Lamentations 3:18, 21, 25-26 and 29 tell us about hope in the Lord.

Please write down a few lessons you can learn about hope from Lamentations.

____

____

____

____

As Christians we have a hope in Jesus Christ our Savior. This hope endures through good times and bad—a hope that originates from God and that remains under all circumstances.

The habit of solitude

After this experience, I grew to appreciate the spiritual discipline of solitude and sought out times to practice it. Yet living in a college dorm room with two roommates rarely provided the opportunity.

One afternoon my roommates were gone, so I pulled out my stethoscope and sat on my bed listening to my the gurgle of my intestines. I re-read Lamentations and praised God for His salvation and the hope He provided.

In the midst of a beautiful moment of solitude, my door flew open; one of my roommates burst in the room. She stopped mid-step and asked, "What are you doing!?!?" I could tell she expected to find an empty room. To find her roommate with a stethoscope and a Bible only added to her shock. To fill the awkward silence, I tried to explain my moment of solitude. She gave me a weird look and quickly left the room.

This past year I reminisced with that roommate about college days. We discussed how we both were very different with the exception of following Christ. She laughed and mentioned that day she burst in the room. From that moment on she classified me as a "little strange."

Everyone may not understand your practice of the spiritual discipline of solitude. However, it allows you to give priority time to God, your hope and salvation.

Life swings like a pendulum from trials to times of ease and excitement. I encourage you in every stage of life to seek the Lord through the practice of solitude.

Today please mediate on God's Word and spend time in prayer but this time, make sure you do it in solitude. Go to a place where you are alone. If you struggle to find a time, try early morning or late evening.

Take a moment to think about the place you will go to practice solitude. It doesn't have to be glamorous—just realistic. Below write down your plan.

____

____

Please read Hebrews 6:13-20 as a reminder.

Day 1 Health Bite

"Don, slow down!" was the persistent plea I heard at the family dinner table as I grew up.

Do you eat as if the food may jump off the plate? Are you "present" when you eat? Or are you distracted by the TV or children? Do you multi-task? Being "mindful" and purposeful when you eat can have a tremendous effect on weight and enjoyment of food, as it allows increased awareness of portion size and flavor. Too often we mindlessly eat and fail to set aside time to fully enjoy and appreciate food. Only in America do we see a person eating a burger and fries while the person walks down the street!

Strategies to master mindful eating

1. Turn off the TV or computer. Eat at the table with your family or listen to relaxing music.
2. Avoid eating out of a box, bag, or container. All food must be on a plate!
3. Make a point of knowing where your produce comes from—this may aid in greater appreciation. (That apple was picked off a tree just for you!) This can serve as an education lesson for your children.
4. Create a fun atmosphere at mealtime; use colorful napkins or plates!
5. Chew foods well; notice the flavor and texture.
6. Ban "desk" eating at work and home. Find a friend with whom you can eat, or take lunch to the local park!

Practicing "mindful eating" not only is good for your health, but it will offer more opportunity to quiet your heart and mind to spend time with the Lord.

This week I will practice "mindful eating" in the following way(s):

____

____

____

Week 5 - Day 2

Jesus, an Example in Solitude

Memory Verse:

"Then Haggai, the Lord's messenger, gave this message of the Lord to the people: 'I am with you,' declares the Lord" (Hag. 1:13).

Our goal as Christians is to follow Christ's example. Therefore our study of solitude remains incomplete without looking at Jesus' practice of this discipline.

Please turn in your Bible to the first gospel and read Matthew 14:1-36.

Jesus Christ is fully God and fully human, but in the Bible story he still takes time out of His busy ministry schedule to commune with God in solitude. As mere human beings we, too, can benefit from taking time to practice the discipline of solitude and seeking the Lord.

Jesus seeks solitude amid what two circumstances? Read the following passages and fill in the blanks below.

1) After John the Baptist's d________. (Matt. 14:13)
   • Solitude can occur after a significant event.
2) In the middle of a busy teaching s___________. (Matt. 14:23)
   • You can practice solitude while you keep up a busy life.

Marking a significant event

Matthew tells us how Jesus practices solitude after He hears about John's death. In life, we encounter many significant events. By practicing solitude at these times we can debrief in the presence and counsel of our Holy and Loving God.

Why wait for tragedy or suffering? A birthday represents the exciting start of another year and the mark of another significant event in our lives. Several years ago, after I studied Matthew 14 and other passages, I formed a new tradition. Around my birthday I try to take one evening and practice the discipline of solitude.

These evenings help me to refocus my life and assess whether my daily activities line up with my mission statement. But more important than the personal evaluation, doing this helps me to learn more about the heart of my Heavenly Father and to develop a greater understanding of my Savior.

Kangarooing

I typically work as an outpatient dietitian. However, occasionally I like to help out on the inpatient floors. Two years ago my birthday fell on a weekday when I was scheduled to work in the neonatal intensive care unit (NICU). I love to occasionally go and work with the little babies. They are precious and so tiny. The diapers have about a three-inch width; some of the babies practically fall out of them.

These tiny babies usually have numerous tubes for feeding, breathing, and medications. They need continuous care. Occasionally the babies have a break from the constant flutter of health professionals and get a chance to bond with their parents. In the NICU they call this *kangarooing*. For about an hour each parent can go in and hold his or her baby. The nurses gently place the baby skin-to-skin with Mom or Dad. The baby appears to be stuck down the parent's shirt. This allows the child to bond with the parent, smell the parent's scent, and feel his or her warmth.

On my commute home that day I thought about things I needed to do before my time of solitude with God. And this reminded me about the preparation that takes place before a parent arrives to "kangaroo". Just like those babies, I benefited from time of bonding with my heavenly Father.

When was the last time you set aside to bond with God?

So, how do you fit this spiritual discipline into a busy schedule? You plan for it. Here are just a few ideas:

- **Yearly solitude:** Seek out a day or an evening (example: birthday) to pray and seek the Lord. Seek His will and reflect to see whether your current life stage and direction line up with what God has revealed to you.
- **Weekly solitude:** Take a Sabbath day of rest. This does not have to occur on Saturday or Sunday, but choose a day or part of a day in which you seek the Lord alone. For example, after a Bible study with other believers, practice the discipline of solitude by reflecting on the lesson and how God may want you to apply His truth to your life.
- **Daily solitude:** This can be as simple as your quiet time. The Scripture says Jesus went off by Himself to pray. For the first two years out of college I had approximately an hour commute to work. The best time for me to seek solitude and pray was in the car during my commute. Numerous times God allowed the moments of solitude and prayer to help me focus on His will.

For several years after he accepted Christ, the apostle Paul spent time away from the crowds. He represents a frequently mentioned example of an individual seeking time alone with God to grow closer to Christ.

Please read Galatians 1:11-24 and meditate on the impact this time had on Paul.

Day 2 Health Bite

As the church family helps to hold its members accountable and then restores them to fellowship when they stray, each of us needs to help each other stay as healthy as we can be.

So take a minute and look back at your initial health inventory and see how you are progressing. How are you doing? To succeed, let your desire for success be greater than your fear of failure. One of our favorite verses is Philippians 4:13 (NASB): *I can do everything through him who gives me strength.*

The marathon is a long way to run. Twenty-six miles is the distance from my home to the neighboring town in which I attended a community college. I drove this distance daily as an impatient commuter. I later began to think of this distance as I began a running program for my personal fitness. As I increased my daily mileage and joined a running club that sponsored races every Saturday morning, I became more excited about the possibility of a marathon, which is 26 miles.

I developed a weekly schedule of varying distances and intensities. This made little "deposits" into the training bank. Those deposits continued to build and build until the big day.

That special day featured great weather and was ideal for the anticipated "withdrawal" of all those months of training "deposits." The feeling of accomplishment was great; I continued to run many more marathons.

The BMI (Body Mass Index) is a commonly used indicator of body composition. Height and weight are used to calculate the BMI. Use the "Body Mass Index Chart" (page 185) in the appendix to calculate your BMI.

Challenge: Walk 45 minutes.
Do 10 push-ups.
Do 30 crunches.

Week 5 - Day 3

The Discipline of Simplicity

Memory Verse:

"Then Haggai, the Lord's messenger, gave this message of the Lord to the people: 'I am with you,' declares the Lord" (Hag. 1:13).

Today we begin our study of the spiritual discipline of simplicity. As we mentioned in the lesson, simplicity boils down to intentionally living to please the Lord. Our primary passage for the study of simplicity is from the book of Haggai.

Please turn to and read Haggai 1.

Haggai's target audience

The first verse of Haggai provides us with very important contextual information. Fill in the blanks with the information you find in this verse.

When was this book written? ______________________________

List the four people mentioned and their jobs.
1) ______________________________
2) ______________________________
3) ______________________________
4) ______________________________

Haggai begins by announcing *in the second year of King Darius*. Who is King Darius? ______________________________

Why does Haggai use the Persian calendar to mark his message? Further, why would a Jewish man writing to a Jewish audience living in Jerusalem mention a foreign king as his first contextual clue? He does this because King Darius of Persia ruled at the time.[1]

The Jews are a conquered people—originally conquered by Babylon. Darius' predecessor, King Cyrus of Persia, conquers Babylon and combines both countries into the Persian Empire.[2] Moved by God, Cyrus issues an edict that the Jewish exiles return home and rebuild the Temple. Yet, many still live in Persia as exiles.

Haggai addresses the remnant of Jews living in war-torn Jerusalem. These Jews intend to rebuild the Temple. Thus Haggai stands as our first postexilic prophet. Based on Babylonian and Jewish records historians have determined Haggai brought this message from the Lord 18 years after the exiled Jews had returned home.[3]

Governor and high priest

God sends a message for the people about His unfinished temple. Yet, Haggai mentions that the Lord sends the message specifically to Zerubbabel and Joshua, the two influential leaders covering both government and religious activities.

Do you currently serve in a position of leadership? Have you in the past? If so, describe the position.

____

____

If God gives a message to you through His Word, how do you respond?

____

____

____

Time for worship

God sends this message to His people during a religious festival—possibly the New Moon festival, a monthly religious celebration meant as a time to break from work, worship in God's house, and listen to a Word from God.[4]

The name Haggai uses to refer to the Lord is the *Lord Almighty* or the *Lord of Hosts*. The word for *hosts* in the Hebrew literally means: "the Almighty, with a focus on great power to conquer or rule."[5]

How significant that God refers to Himself as the *Lord of Hosts—the Lord Almighty* to the remnant who meet to worship alongside the unfinished temple. Maybe the people feel overwhelmed and powerless to accomplish the task. Yet they are there to worship the Almighty God.

Simplicity and reality

A life of simplicity—how wonderful and peaceful it sounds! Yet how close to reality does it seem? Yes, a life of simplicity—one of complete devotion to the Lord in all aspects of life—may be your heart's desire. Yet I feel sure that you struggle with implementing this discipline. I do.

Today God has a message for us. The first thing to know is that He is the Lord Almighty, Lord of Hosts! He has the power to conquer and reign in our lives.

Take time to meditate on your Lord Almighty. What difference does knowing God as the Lord of Hosts make to you? Describe.

____

____

The Message

Haggai begins his message with a prophetic statement: *This is what the Lord Almighty says: "Give careful thought to your ways."* Twice in Haggai we find this exact phrase.

The challenge the Lord gives His people is to consider their ways. Evaluate your life, He says. Haggai continues with the Lord's message

> *You have planted much, but harvested little.*
> *You eat, but never have enough.*
> *You drink, but never have your fill.*
> *You put on clothes, but are not warm.*
> *You earn wages, only to put them in a purse with holes in it.*

Do you sense that God's message for the remnant applies to you? Could He ask the same and it prove true? No matter how diligently you work, no matter what you plan, it just doesn't meet your needs. It does not satisfy.

We don't find Haggai bringing the typical prophetic message—*repent of your sin and return to the Lord.*[6] Instead he asks the people about their work. These investments they seek and that they labor and toil to get have turned up lacking. God asks the people to question the pace and purpose of their lives. What about us? Have we poured our work, time, and resources into worthy investments?

The God of our provision

In Haggai 1:7-11, again the Lord of Hosts asks His people to consider their ways. Now He brings them back to their job assignments for the last 18 years. They return home to rebuild the Lord's temple, yet it sits unfinished while they busy themselves with other work.

How about your life? Has God given you a job assignment? How close are you to finishing it?

____

____

____

Has God challenged you to get involved at your church? Has God encouraged you to pray regularly with your family?

____

____

In Haggai 1:7-11, we find that God states He has taken away their gain from the crops and labor since they seek their own personal pursuits without obeying the Lord and building the temple. Take a moment and meditate on this concept.

Do you ever think the Lord may have let you feel the consequences of going your own way? Or the Lord Almighty may have blown away the gain so that we may become dissatisfied with our pursuits to help us recognize our lack of obedience.

Responding with obedience

Then Zerubbabel son of Shealtiel and Joshua son of Jehozadak, the high priest, with all the remnant of the people [who had returned from captivity], listened to and obeyed the voice of the Lord their God [not vaguely or partly, but completely, according to] the words of Haggai the prophet, since the Lord their God had sent him, and the people [reverently] feared and [worshipfully] turned to the Lord (Hag. 1:12 Amplified).

Please read Haggai 1:12-15. If you could choose two words to describe the remnant's response, what would you write? ____________________ and

____

Here we see an immediate response to a message from God. Haggai tells us that the whole remnant obeys. It starts with the leaders, but everyone chooses to act. Very soon the people diligently began to work on the temple.

Haggai 1:13 gives another message to the remnant. What Word does God send to His people?

____

____

The promise of God's presence is enough to motivate them to work. I don't know whether today you are frustrated or enthusiastic about the work God has given you. You already may practice the spiritual discipline of simplicity. But regardless where we are, the promise of God's presence is enough to stir our ___________________ (excited, frustrated, lazy, or weary—you fill in the blank) hearts so that we will live completely devoted to Him.

I appreciate the remnant and Haggai for this message of hope. It is a hope that when we align ourselves with the Lord's will, He reminds us of His presence and still is willing to use us. After 18 years the people again seek to honor the Lord by building His Temple.

You may have taken a detour in your relationship with God. But today you can recommit your life to singleheartedly following Christ. This commitment will change what you think, say, and do. It will impact your schedule and resources. But knowing that the Lord is with you makes following Him peaceful and satisfying.

King Solomon writes the book of Ecclesiastes. He basks in fame during his reign and pursues many avenues to bring him meaning, pleasure, and satisfaction. Yet in the end he finds that without God he remains dissatisfied.

Please read the book of Ecclesiastes. Meditate on how to apply the spiritual discipline of simplicity in your own life.

Day 3 Health Bite

Research is clear—certain foods help prevent disease. Your food choices today will most likely influence your future. If you want to take steps to protect your heart and mind, several times this week make a conscious effort to include these five "disease fighters".

1. Salmon and Tuna: These are rich in omega-3 fatty acids that fight inflammation. Studies show a diet high in omega-3s may reduce heart disease by 30 to 40 percent. Try to eat at least three servings (1 serving = 4 ounces) of one of the omega-3 rich fish each week. (Choose chunk light tuna and wild salmon most often.)
2. Blueberries: The blueberry is packed with fiber, Vitamin C, and is one of the richest foods in antioxidants. Toss on cereal, eat as a snack, or enjoy frozen with low-fat milk for a refreshing treat!
3. Beans and Oatmeal: Both are an excellent source of soluble fiber, which helps eliminate unhealthy cholesterol. Beans (especially pinto, lima, navy, black, kidney) are easy to prepare and can be served as a side dish or tossed in salads, soups, and stir-fry's or on nachos! Start the day with a bowl of oatmeal several days a week or try one for a snack.
4. Ground Flaxseed: It is a rich plant source of omega-3 fatty acids and fiber! Try using 1 to 2 tablespoons ground flaxseed daily. Sprinkle on yogurt, salads, or stews, or add to muffins and sweet breads.
5. Broccoli: Broccoli is rich in Vitamin C, folate, and soluble fiber, which help fight high cholesterol and cancer. Eat it raw with low-fat dip or steamed or sautéed with a squeeze of lemon and fresh ground pepper.

My plan this week to protect my heart with disease-fighting foods:

____

____

____

____

Week 5 - Day 4

A Case of Comparing

Memory Verse:

"Then Haggai, the Lord's messenger, gave this message of the Lord to the people: 'I am with you,' declares the Lord" (Hag. 1:13).

Today we find ourselves in Haggai 2:1-9. For approximately a month the remnant has worked on rebuilding the temple.[1] We find God's people benefiting from another Word from God.

God sends a message to the remnant. He asks the people three questions (Hag. 2:3).
1) *Who of you is left who saw this house in its former glory?*
2) *How does it look to you now?*
3) *Does it not seem to you like nothing?*

These questions reveal that He understands their circumstance and challenges. He hears their frustration and complaints about the new temple.

Why the comparison and complaining? The remnant has received clearance from a foreign king to go home and work. God has obviously opened an opportunity and a means to complete the temple. He also gives the people a promise of His presence. What more do they need?

Yet, sometime within the first month, the remnant starts to compare. The people begin to compare the temple to its predecessor—the one King Solomon built. Solomon and the Israelites have constructed a magnificent temple. In its construction they use gold, silver, bronze, wood, and beautifully embroidered linen. (For more information on the first temple, please read 1 Kings 1-11.) "*The temple I am going to build will be great, because our God is greater than all other gods*" (2 Chron. 2:5).

Be strong and work

In Haggai the Lord gives a message for His people that will cure their discouragement and motivate them to obey. This new message from the Lord is a call to action—a call to follow through and finish the task. "*Be strong . . . and work*" (Hag. 2:4).

What about you? Do you understand the sentiments of the Israelites as they compare their work to those before them? Do you ever take an assessment and conclude that your work lacks the grandeur, perceived significance, or glory?

How can we find the strength to be strong and work? I believe God in Haggai 2:4-5 tells of the source of the remnant's strength: "*For I am with you . . . my Spirit remains among you. Do not fear.*"

When you face obstacles and struggle with the temptation to give up, remember your Lord Almighty. His presence in your life will be the source of your strength. As you practice the discipline of simplicity, you can learn from these three encouragements from the Lord: 1) recognize the presence of God, the Lord Almighty; 2) be strong; and 3) work.

A future glory

God then provides a message foretelling a future event. Please read Haggai 2:6-9. Answer the following questions.

What does God tell us about Himself?

____

____

What does He tell His people about the temple?

____

____

Greater glory

The glimmer of gold and brilliance of bronze bring beauty, but what brings glory to the temple of God? Please read 2 Chronicles 7:1-3; write down what brings glory to Solomon's temple.

____

____

A breathtaking flash of fire and the glory of the Lord descends on the temple. Chronicles' historical account tells that the glory of the first temple arrives with God's presence.

In Haggai, the Lord's first message is a promise of His presence. The people complain when the temple does not meet their expectations. Yet, God's presence determines the glory of a place.

The people of the remnant struggle in their work because they focus on the outward beauty of the temple instead of on God's glory. Here we find in Haggai one temptation to quit the practice of simplicity. A life of simplicity does not guarantee us a life of glamour or prestige. If we allow possessions, relationships, or responsibilities to distract us from following the Lord with complete devotion, then we have forsaken the practice of simplicity.

But God does more than just remind this remnant that the glory of the temple springs from His presence. He tells the people that the temple they work to build will have a greater glory.

One day God does bring greater glory to this temple. This temple remains standing during Jesus' lifetime.[2] Jesus Christ, the One, true God in human flesh, walks and teaches in the temple courts (Luke 2:41-52 and Luke 19:45-20:8).

In the book of Proverbs, we find a prayer of simplicity. Today please read Proverbs 30:7-9. Meditate on the motives behind this prayer.

Day 4 Health Bite

Homework: Apples vs. Pears

Motivation: Success—what you do with what you've got.

Assignment: The distribution of body fat in the abdomen, chest, and lower back increases the risk for heart disease, stroke, type II diabetes, and some forms of cancer. This fat accumulation is known as the **"apple shape."** Fat that gathers in the hips, buttocks, and thighs is commonly called the **"pear shape."** Ideally, your hips should be larger than your waist. "Pears" are at lower risk than "apples" are. Assess your risk following the instructions on the "Hip-to-Waist Ratio" on page 186 in the appendix.

Challenge: Walk 50 minutes.
Do 10 push-ups.
Do 30 crunches.

Verse: *He energizes those who get tired, gives fresh strength to dropouts. For even young people tire and drop out, young folk in their prime stumble and fall. But those who wait upon God get fresh strength. They spread their wings and soar like eagles. They run and don't get tired, they walk and don't lag behind* (Isa. 40:30-31 The Message).

Week 5 - Day 5

Cookie Nights

Memory Verse:

"Then Haggai, the Lord's messenger, gave this message of the Lord to the people: 'I am with you,' declares the Lord" (Hag. 1:13).

During my freshman year in college a small group of my friends began staging habitual "cookie nights". We occasionally met together to chat, for encouragement, and to eat. By the name of the occasion, you can tell we placed an emphasis on food.

Our cookie nights usually were spontaneous. Once we determined a time and place, we appointed a few people to bring in the loot for our enjoyment. A cookie cake or ice cream usually fit the bill.

One morning after a cookie night I attended a nutrition class in which we studied in detail eating disorders. Before the class I completed my reading without applying any of the information to real life. However, in class I sat surprised at the realization I made. On closer inspection, I determined that I was a *group binge-eater*. The thought shocked me so much that I turned to my classmate on my left and confessed my involvement in cookie nights. She, too, admitted her tendency to overeat, especially when she was around a few of her Christian friends.

Before that day, I did not think we had a problem. The class discussion got me thinking that a better way must exist. Yet I did not make any life changes; I considered this awareness to be only "food for thought".

A couple of years later as our cookie nights continued; one of my friends in the group approached me for help. She noticed weight gain and found eating correctly alongside our habit to be challenging. Since I was the only nutrition major in the group, she jokingly chided me on my bad influence.

That day we devised a plan to change the cookie night to a fruit night. The next time this group got together, the two of us purchased delicious fruit, washed, sliced, and aesthetically arranged the fruit on a platter. We ended our evening with only a quarter of the plate devoured; we realized how differently the evening went when we took the focus off food. Did we have genuine fellowship? Yes. For that night we sought to build up the body of Christ both spiritually and physically. In hindsight, I realized that fellowship can and does continue even when you alter its relationship with food.

Do you have any traditions with others that encourage unhealthy lifestyle habits?

____

____

____

If you do, please take a moment and write down a realistic alteration to your less-than-healthy tradition.

____

____

____

The purpose of this study is to help people of the church serve the Lord at optimum capacity. We seek to provide you practical tools as you seek to glorify God with your spiritual and physical health. Yet through personal study I recognize the relationship between the two.

What is gluttony?

Gluttony, according to Merriam-Webster, is "1: excess in eating or drinking and 2: greedy or excessive indulgence"(*http://www.merriam-webster.com/dictionary/gluttony 10/13/07*).

From Scripture I find warnings against gluttony and descriptions of the consequences.

Please look up and read Proverbs 23:20-21.

Gluttony is one factor leading to poverty and drowsiness. We see here that gluttony can steal from one's resources: money and energy.

Please look up and read Amos 5 and 6.

Amos is a prophet previously employed as a shepherd from Tekoa. God sends him from Judah to preach a message of judgment to Israel. He first tells of judgment on Israel's neighbors and then brings the message home. The temptation to care for ourselves above others can have an influence on our health.

How did the Israelites' selfishness influence those around them?

____

____

But Amos preaches the Lord's message—His solution, besides identifying their sin of selfishness and complacency. *This is what the Lord says to the house of Israel: "Seek me and live; do not seek Bethel, do not go to Gilgal, do not journey to Beersheba. For Gilgal will surely go into exile, and Bethel will be reduced to nothing. Seek the Lord and live, or he will sweep through the house of Joseph like a fire; it will devour, and Bethel will have no one to quench it*" (Amos 5:4-6).

Amos brings a message of repentance—a call to wake up from the people's lethargic apathy and to live intentionally, thus bringing about the purpose of the Lord here on earth. That requires good stewardship of the energy and resources God provides them.

Abundance

Those of us in the Western world live in a time of affluence and plenty. Poverty and hunger do occur in our society, but overall we cannot compare ourselves to the hunger and need in Third World countries. Practicing the spiritual discipline of simplicity requires recognizing God as provider and owner of all our resources. Let us be good managers of what God has given and not allow the food, which God intended to provide nourishment and enjoyment, to become our drug of choice and prevent us from living life completely surrendered to God's will and work. Instead, let us use our resources and energy to further the kingdom of God.

As believers, we live to love God and others. If I do everything in my power to live a strong, healthy life, then I can serve the Lord as long and diligently as physically possible. This desire and decision influences my daily life. It impacts my eating and exercise habits. For example:
1) When I meet with friends who want to lose weight, my goal is to encourage them to make healthier choices. I accomplish this first by choosing healthier foods myself.
2) Other times a friend may struggle with an eating disorder. I intentionally eat a food the person would classify as unhealthy and off-limits.

Occasionally in life we have no control over the circumstances. Yet, regarding our health, the average person has a significant amount of control. Personal responsibility accompanies that. Overall, my goal is to encourage everyone to serve the Lord at his or her greatest capacity. This means letting our allegiance to God dictate our view of and motivation for health. The culture and our circumstances often provide obstacles along the way. However, by the grace and love of God we have the strength to continue on and to work to accomplish our goals about our spiritual and physical health.

Please read 1 Corinthians 8:1-13. Meditate on the role of food in the life of a believer.

Day 5 Health Bite

Stress and sleep. Both can have a profound effect on your weight, energy level, and quality of life. Why? Research seems to show a strong link between weight gain and inadequate sleep and high stress. This could be for various reasons. First, a hormone imbalance may result; that imbalance causes an increase in weight gain around the midsection. Second, fatigue may lead to increased food intake and less "mindfulness" when eating, while stress may lead to emotional eating.

Professionals agree that adults are to aim for at least seven to nine hours of sleep per night. I have observed how improved sleeping habits and stress-reduction directly affects weight loss.

Evaluate your sleep and stress. If one or the other needs improvement, take some time over the weekend to think about how you may need to make sleep or stress management a priority. Professional counseling can be an excellent resource to assist with strategies to manage stress. If you suspect a sleep disorder, talk with your healthcare professional to determine possible therapies.

On average how much sleep do you get? ______________________________

On a scale of (low) 1-10 (high) how would you rate your stress level?

____

Goals:

I will get _______ hours of sleep at least _______ times next week.

I will try to bring my stress level down from a level ______ to a level ______ by ____.

**Remember to take your concerns to the Lord if you feel overwhelmed by stress or lack of sleep.

**Great Read: *Mindless Eating* by Brian Wansick

Week 6 - Day 1

Time to Party

Memory Verse:

Then Jesus came to them and said, "All authority in heaven and on earth has been given to me. Therefore go and make disciples of all nations, baptizing them in the name of the Father and of the Son and of the Holy Spirit, and teaching them to obey everything I have commanded you. And surely I am with you always, to the very end of the age" (Matt. 28:18-20).

A busy day at work—out of my peripheral vision I spied the clock, quickly finished up a little computer work, and then hurried off to greet my new clients. After I scanned the scene, I saw a delightful couple. We made polite introductions; I escorted them back to my office to begin the session.

Early on the wife stated, "I think we should tell you something. You see . . . we like to celebrate . . . frequently . . . and we do it with food."

"What constitutes a celebration?" I asked

"Oh . . . a bright sunny day, a difficult day at work, an anniversary . . ." (she sank a glance at her husband and smiled) ". . . anything," she said with a ring in her voice.

"Can you help?" she asked hesitantly.

"Of course!" I said.

Although I haven't met with that husband and wife for a while now, I remember their joy and keenness for parties. As Christians we, too, have many reasons and celebrate at every stage in life. Today I want us to look in the gospel of Luke; Jesus taught us about rejoicing in heaven.

Today we begin our study on the spiritual discipline of evangelism. Please read Luke 15:1-7.

A hopeless cause

Luke 15 tells the story of the lost sheep, coin, and son. This chapter is a favorite because of its beautiful description of God's love and forgiveness.

To understand the context for these stories please read Luke 15:1-2.

From this verse we can find a variety of people who listen to Jesus' teaching. First, we find the tax collectors—hated by all. They cheat their own people out of hard-earned wages by charging them more than the Roman government requires. Second, we have "sinners", or those who do not follow the law. Finally we have the Pharisees and religious leaders. Their responsibilities include teaching God's truth found in the laws and the prophets. What a mix! Here we find a group of religious teachers and students who obviously do not apply their message.

These demographics provide fuel for the Pharisees' and religious leaders' criticism of Jesus Christ. Why in the world would a rabbi spend time with religious rejects?

Jesus has a different view of those considered hopeless and unholy. He loves them and teaches them about repentance and salvation—a message many of the self-righteous religious leaders refuse to receive.

In response, Jesus tells them a parable—a story about a great love, a search, a restoration, and of course, a party!

The heart of our Savior

Please read Luke 15:3-7. Fill in the spaces below.

How does the shepherd view the sheep?

____

____

How does this perspective influence the shepherd's actions?

____

In the end, Jesus mentions rejoicing in heaven. What does this reveal about the character of God?

____

____

In these five verses, I believe we find a Word from God's heart about the practice of evangelism. We find a loving, forgiving God who seeks out those who do not follow Him. The shepherd does not wait for the lost sheep to arrive at its senses. The shepherd pursues the sheep. In the same way evangelism involves going out to seek out those who do not know this God of love.

How do we know the target audience of this verse? This parable at first may seem like a story of a believer who takes a brief detour in following Christ. Yet, the listeners consist of Jews—God's chosen people. Jesus teaches that each person needs to choose to follow Him for salvation (John 14:6). We have a message given to God's chosen people, the Jews, who personally reject Him; this includes the tax collectors, sinners, and religious leaders.[1]

Today we also have a Word from God, found in the Holy Bible, about salvation. We have the same choice. Will we accept or reject Christ?

Think about your family, friends, and acquaintances. Who are *the lost sheep*?

____

____

How does this parable influence your relationship with them?

____

Here we find a foundational element for the practice of evangelism. It requires the compassion and love of your Savior. It requires going to those outside of the church and bringing them the Truth about Jesus. Will you share God's love, hope, and salvation with the world?

Time to party!

The clients I mentioned earlier had an affinity for celebrations. What about you? In this passage, Jesus tells us that all of heaven rejoices when just one person repents of his or her sin and turns to follow Christ. Take a moment and think about this concept. I have no grasp on the beauty, the majesty, or the enormity of heaven. I have difficulty conceiving that when you, your friends or family, or anyone anywhere in the world becomes a Christian, all of heaven rejoices.

This parable brings to light God's love for each person. As long as a person has life, that person is not a lost cause. Jesus Christ, the Good Shepherd, is sent to restore sinners. He is Truth. We can trust in His teaching, accept the forgiveness He offers, and give Him our lives.

We know the Good Shepherd! Therefore we have reason to rejoice every day. Today spend some time praying about your practice of evangelism. Pray that God will give you a heart that resembles His. Keep your eyes open to the lost sheep He wants you to go after with a message of hope, love, and forgiveness.

Today take time to think about the lost in your life. Maybe you know a person or group of people that some consider religious rejects. Today spend time praying for them. Seek to reach out to them soon. Consider sharing with your accountability partner or group the names of lost sheep. Think of ways that you as a group can reach out and share God's love and hope.

Please read Matthew 9:9-13.

Day 1 Health Bite

Food only—or are supplements necessary? More than one-third of all Americans report that they regularly take a multivitamin/mineral supplement (MVI). A study by the National Institute of Health found that MVI users saved $8 billion per year in health-care costs compared to nonusers. However, the research is not clear whether these supplements actually can protect us from specific diseases. Studies do show that people who take a daily MVI report feeling healthier and have more energy. One of the primary reasons to consider taking a MVI is to supplement nutrients you fail to obtain from your diet. Most Americans do not meet all necessary nutritional needs on a daily basis. Multivitamins may be particularly important for women and the elderly.

We live in a culture that looks for the "latest and greatest" cure for all our ailments and that helps us lose weight and provides more energy. Too often we fail to focus on the proven remedy for a healthy lifestyle—a varied, well-balanced eating and exercise plan. Food is the most effective way to obtain nutrients. An MVI will not meet all your nutritional needs; make food choices the primary focus! Think of your MVI as your "insurance policy" for obtaining optimal health!

Tips:

1. Research studies suggest higher-cost supplements do not necessarily provide a higher quality or have advantages over lower-cost generic brand preparations.
2. When possible choose a supplement that has the USP (United States Pharmacopeia) symbol on the bottle. (This may help ensure that the supplement's nutritional claims are more accurate.)
3. Take your MVI with food if it tends to make you nauseated or hungry, or take it after dinner or bedtime.
4. Take your MVI around the same time every day to help you remember.

**Additional supplements (vitamin, mineral, herbal) may be useful to assist with disease management and/or prevention. However, this must be determined on an individual basis. Discuss supplements with your physicians, registered dietitian, or nutritionist to determine what may be best for you. Always consult with a physician before you begin any new vitamin, mineral, or herbal supplement.

Week 6 - Day 2

My Herb Garden

Memory Verse:

Then Jesus came to them and said, "All authority in heaven and on earth has been given to me. Therefore go and make disciples of all nations, baptizing them in the name of the Father and of the Son and of the Holy Spirit, and teaching them to obey everything I have commanded you. And surely I am with you always, to the very end of the age" (Matt. 28:18-20).

Did you know I have a garden? Makes sense, right? I am a dietitian. You might assume that my training taught me a little bit about agriculture. And it did.

Yet, interest with a little knowledge does not constitute skill. You see, I lack a green thumb. A couple of my roommates knew how to take care of plants and herbs. While we roomed together, they kept quite a few plants alive. As they married off, they left the plants in my care—in hindsight, a horrible thing to do. To my own shame I have even killed a cactus.

Each year I try a different technique for gardening. To make matters more difficult, I live in an apartment complex without a balcony and with minimal sunlight. However, this year I think I have got it. And with pride I tell you that all of the herbs have sprouts. Yeah! I am off to a good start.

What is my secret? Well . . . for Christmas my parents gave me an indoor herb garden. This garden contains its own irrigation system and lighting. I occasionally fill a vat with water, drop in a few nutrient pills, and when ready, harvest the herbs. How wonderful—perfect for the busy city-dweller who cannot seem to keep a plant alive! You see, I have minimal investment and maximum results.

This week we study the spiritual discipline of evangelism. We will look at a passage in which God compares the practice of evangelism with a harvest. On closer inspection of this passage I recognize that my experience with gardening would not provide a proper understanding of God's Word. I do not know what your experience with evangelism or harvesting has been. But today for the sake of understanding this passage, please try to put aside your perspectives and arrive fresh to this study of evangelism. See whether He will change your perspective as He has mine.

The compassion component

Please read Matthew 9:35-38. Please take a moment and meditate on verse 36.

In this verse we find two facts important for the practice of evangelism. First, we have a God of compassion. Our God sees the condition of all and hears their cries of help. When you practice evangelism, follow our Lord's example. Have compassion for those around the world.

Second, recognize that many do not know truth. Because of this they are vulnerable to false teachers and to the consequences of sin. They have not heard of a loving God who offers them salvation and a new way of life.

As Christ-followers who seek to practice evangelism, we often find that the first step is to recognize the need. For example, as English-speakers we have access to the Bible, God's inspired Word. Yet in our world we have more than 2,200 language communities who do not have a copy of the Bible. That adds up to approximately 200-million people.[1]

Begin with prayer

Prayer exists as a vital component of evangelism. In Matthew 9, Jesus instructs His disciples to pray.

How does He want them to pray?

____

____

He prays that people would volunteer to go and serve. The need exists. But occasionally we allow life to interfere with this discipline. We become too busy and forget about the lost around the world. Whether or not you practice evangelism regularly, a good place to start is with prayer

Intentional life

Evangelism may seem natural when you are on a mission trip across the ocean. However, what about back at home? One lesson that mission trips have taught me is to live intentionally. I try to apply to daily life four tips I picked up from missionaries. I find by including these four things I am more likely to intentionally seek to share about Christ.

1) Read about other cultures, communities, and religions.
Go to your church library and read books about other cultures and religions. Specifically compare a religion's sacred works, deities, mode of salvation, teachings on morality, and belief about afterlife. Meet with your accountability partner and together discuss the differences.

In high school, I began studying other faiths to see what they believed. I started the search with a few friends as a project at church. In our small Acteens group, a missions organization, we would return to present on our assigned religion and compare it to Christianity. In the end, it helped to articulate my faith to friends at school who followed other religions. It allowed me to discuss the important issues and not to argue. The time spent studying helped us to practice the discipline of evangelism.

2) Regularly pray for witnessing opportunities.
Plan a consistent time for prayer. Put it on your calendar and assign specific individuals a day of the week. Remember to consistently pray for them.

3) Listen to the Holy Spirit. When you sense His guidance, share the good news.
We find numerous biblical examples of how the Holy Spirit guides Christians to share the gospel. As a result, the New Testament church grows. I look back and regrettably realize that too many times I remained silent. My prayer for all of us is a listening ear and the boldness to speak the truth.

4) Maintain relationships!
Remember that God calls a person to Himself (John 16:5-16). You do not win a soul based on your evangelism technique. We follow God's example of going, sharing, and above all, loving. I believe people can tell when we truly love them. This love compels us to share the truth we know. Regardless whether they accept or reject Christ, our response is to remain consistent: pray, go, share, and of course, love.

If you ask a farmer about his harvest, you likely would hear of an incredible personal investment—very different than my experience with herbs. In the practice of evangelism, God challenges us to invest in the lives of others. The practice of this discipline ultimately requires maximum investment with a complete trust in God about the results of the harvest.

Please take time to read Isaiah 6:1-13 and 1 Corinthians 13:1-13. Take time to meditate on these passages in light of our study of evangelism.

How has God challenged you to help with the harvest?

____

____

____

Day 2 Health Bite

Accept the challenge so that you may feel the exhilaration of victory. Enhanced muscular strength and endurance can lead to improvements in the areas of performance, injury prevention, body composition, and lifetime muscle and bone health.

For the muscles and muscle groups to be strengthened, they must be subjected to greater than normal workloads that challenge the muscular system. If one only lifts pens, eating utensils, books, and other light objects, the muscles do very little. However, if the muscles are asked to lift a 15-pound weight 10 times, the muscles are suddenly called on to do a greater task. If this task is repeated over several weeks at regular intervals, the muscle will respond by increasing in strength and size. This principle is the foundation of weight training.

A workout program is a challenge. In fact, that's part of the benefit. It's a challenge because it requires a lot from us. It demands discipline, diligent effort, time, and energy—the very things that often are in short supply. Do it anyway! Then the real value begins to shine through—that of commitment, accomplishment, improved health, stronger self-esteem, and a better quality of life. These are the reasons that we have stuck with a workout program for many years. Some of our favorite motivating verses are: *She makes her arms strong* (Prov. 31:17 NASB), *Whatever you find to do with your hands, do it with all your might* (Eccl. 9:10), and *And that about wraps it up. God is strong and He wants you strong* (Eph. 6:10 The Message).

Challenge: Walk 55 minutes.
Do 12 push-ups.
Do 35 crunches.

Week 6 - Day 3

The Wilton Diptych

Memory Verse:

Then Jesus came to them and said, "All authority in heaven and on earth has been given to me. Therefore go and make disciples of all nations, baptizing them in the name of the Father and of the Son and of the Holy Spirit, and teaching them to obey everything I have commanded you. And surely I am with you always, to the very end of the age" (Matt. 28:18-20).

The summer after my freshman year at college I had the opportunity to study abroad at Christ Church in Oxford with about 15 other college students. For more than a year, my older brother, Brian, had planned to go on this trip. At the last minute I had the opportunity to join him. Of course I jumped at the chance.

For the first week our group stayed in London. Before classes started we spent most of our time visiting tourist attractions. At one of the museums, our group huddled around the Wilton Diptych, a famous painting of a deer lying on a bed of grass. The museum curator spent about five minutes explaining what I understood her to describe as *the heart of this painting* and its significance. I admit that I don't remember exactly what she said. I just stared at the painting and tried to find out what she was talking about, but the meaning seemed nowhere to be found. Finally, I leaned over to Brian and whispered, "Where is the heart?"

Brian paused, shifted, and then whispered back, "Stephanie, . . . it is a picture of a *hart* . . . *H-A-R-T*." Oh . . . then it hit me! Instead of searching for a geometric shape or a smooth muscle, I should have looked for Bambi's father.

I could try to devise an excuse for my ignorance. But truthfully I needed Brian there to explain the difference between *heart* and *hart*—a deer. Otherwise, I remained someone who unknowingly faced the very object I sought.

This week we study the spiritual discipline of evangelism. Today we'll look at Acts 8 and the example of Philip. Philip reminds me of my brother, because he took the time to answer questions and did so in a kind way.

God chooses to use His children to preach and teach the good news about Christ. Today we will study two examples of how to share Christ effectively.

The Ethiopian and the Book of Isaiah

Persecution breaks out in Jerusalem; this leads to the spreading of believers around the world (Acts 8:1). During this time, Philip, an apostle, heads north; he goes to Samaria. All along the way he shares the good news about Jesus and performs miracles. Many people place their faith in Christ and follow His teaching.

In response to the spreading of the gospel, Peter and John arrive from the church in Jerusalem to visit Philip and the new believers in Samaria. The church in Jerusalem represents the mother church or home base for the followers of Christ. Peter and John are leaders. Once they see God's work in people's lives, they head back to Jerusalem.

This is a successful church plant. So now what? Does God tell Philip to drive a stake in the ground and call Samaria home? Surprisingly not; instead God sends another message and tells Philip to go south on a desert road to Gaza (Acts 8:25-26). The message: leave the thriving new flock and travel down a lonely, desert road. Now that presents an interesting turn of events.

Please turn in your Bibles and read Acts 8:26-40. Take a moment to think about this passage. Below summarize how Philip knows where to go and what to do.

____

____

____

On the road Philip sees a high-ranking official in Ethiopia. The man heads home after he worships in Jerusalem. Again we see the Lord direct Philip; he obeys; in Acts 8:29 the Spirit tells Philip to join the chariot.

Philip runs up alongside the chariot to join the official. One thing I appreciate about Philip is his obedience to the Lord's leadership. When Philip gets a Word from God, he does it. He does not linger. He runs.

Philip then hears the eunuch reading from Isaiah; he takes this as his cue to ask a question. The eunuch responds and asks for help.

Have you ever lacked understanding? I appreciate the eunuch's willingness to admit his confusion.

Acts 8:35 tells us how Philip then explains the message of Jesus Christ; he starts with that Scripture passage.

Philip's method provides helpful guidelines when we endeavor to practice the spiritual discipline of evangelism.

1) First, **listen** to the prompting of the Holy Spirit.
2) Then we can willingly **obey** when the Lord leads.
3) Allow the opportunity in front of you to start the **conversation**.
4) Seek to **explain** the gospel and make the message of Christ clear.

Educating Apollos

Now please turn in your Bibles to Acts 18:23-28 and read this passage. Here we find a man who seeks to follow God but lacks the complete gospel. Two Christians befriend him and explain to him the rest of the story.

What similarities do you see between these two instances?

____

____

____

How can you apply these principles to your practice of evangelism?

____

____

Take a moment to meditate on Romans 10:14-15.

Day 3 Health Bite

POW! Are your daily meals filled with enticing flavor and appeal? If not, why not? Meals that taste good and are flavorful and offer more satisfaction and fulfillment. One way to add pizzazz and creativity is to experiment with fresh or dried herbs! Often we view fruits and vegetables as food that offers protection from illness, but surprisingly herbs are packed with their own arsenal of nutritional benefit.

Research suggests the following:

OREGANO: Contains the highest antioxidant activity of all the herbs! It may prevent damage caused by free radicals and boost the immune system.
BASIL: Contains anti-bacterial, anti-fungal, and anti-inflammatory properties.
THYME: Contains the highest antimicrobial activity of all the herbs and may help with chronic and acute bronchitis.
ROSEMARY: Helps to decrease inflammation and may help with peptic ulcers
CINNAMON: May have a role in lowering blood glucose and cholesterol levels when it is used in conjunction with a healthy lifestyle.

How about starting your own herb garden? No matter where you live, for little cost you can plant herbs in pots, containers, or in the ground! Planting herbs may help motivate you to try fresh new recipes. What could be better than stepping out your back door to find fresh basil, oregano, or cilantro?!

If creating your own garden does not sound enchanting, the dried herbs are excellent substitutions. However, herbs loose their nutritional punch if they are stored longer than six months in your pantry.

This week I will add new flavor and pizzazz to my meals by

____

How would you rate your food choices this week? ____ (1=poor; 10=excellent)

How could you make improvements or continue healthy habits?

____

____

Week 6 - Day 4

The Ananias Project

Memory Verse:

Then Jesus came to them and said, "All authority in heaven and on earth has been given to me. Therefore go and make disciples of all nations, baptizing them in the name of the Father and of the Son and of the Holy Spirit, and teaching them to obey everything I have commanded you. And surely I am with you always, to the very end of the age" (Matt. 28:18-20).

In 2002 I had the opportunity to go to Glasgow, Scotland, as a summer missionary. I went to serve as a children's worker at a local Baptist church. When I arrived, I joined a team of three other girls who just started working with youth and refugees about two miles from the church.

We lived in a flat in the housing projects. This experience truly opened my eyes to God's creativity in designing humanity, because in a one-mile radius lived 48 different ethnic groups. I think I was the only Texan. Make that 49 different ethnic groups!

This definitely brought me out of my comfort zone. Like other Americans I remained shocked by the evil of the world around me. September 11th of the previous year stayed fresh in my mind; 2002 was the year two Baylor alumni had been held hostage in Afghanistan.

The first weekend in the flat, my roommates traveled to London to see about a youth program to use as a model for the one they hoped to start. I stayed in Glasgow. This Sunday was my first at the church.

Before I moved in, a well-meaning church member encouraged me to not talk to others because they would know I was not Scottish, not to let anyone know I did not live with a man, and to stay alert. They warned me in this manner because a year beforehand, a stabbing occurred right outside of our apartment complex. *Great!* I thought.

That week I tried to learn my way around Glasgow. The missionary (I'll call her *Fiona*)—the one starting the youth projects program—gave me the job of beginning to plan a prayer walk for mission trips from America that would occur later that summer. That week I wandered around with map in hand. God took complete care of me. In fact, I felt surprisingly safe.

One night I met up with four Scottish college students. We went to see *Spiderman* on opening night. I had already seen it two months before in Texas but was thankful to see familiar faces, so I went along. Afterward they dropped me off at the curb closest to the front door but around at the back of our apartment. So I walk around to the front of our building. There stood a group of refugee men in a huddle by the door. Once I turned the bend, they stopped talking and all turned to look right at me. They stood silent, not moving and not smiling; they were like a cluster of statues blocking the door.

I briefly thought about continuing on my way. Even though I knew little about their culture, I knew not to address men in public, which included not to try to excuse myself as I proceeded through their group.

So I turned back around and ran in the direction I had just traveled. Instead of running like legendary Scottish Olympian Eric Liddell did for the pleasure of God, I ran out of my fear of man. Thankfully in their mirror the other college students saw me and returned. Out of breath, I jumped in the car and asked them to please watch me get safely inside. The two guys in the group kindly returned and walked me through the group of men at the apartment door and watched as I entered the elevator safely.

That night I went back to my flat, got in bed, and prayed. But I could not go to sleep. Above our flat I heard rushing footsteps, angry voices, and pounding. This sounded as though it was a case of domestic abuse. Reality hit home. I was not in Texas anymore!

So I called my parents, an ocean away, and asked them to pray. This probably was not the best thing to do in regard to their comfort, but I longed for their prayers. I had helped with ministry projects before, but this time I felt very alone. God comforted me with His presence (Ps. 34:7).

Soon Fiona and the girls returned from London. I told Fiona about what happened that week and was quite candid about my fears. How do you share about Christ when you do not feel safe enough to go out and meet people?

Fiona mentioned Acts 9, the Scripture passage about Saul's conversion. It tells of Ananias, a disciple from Damascus, who God tells to visit Saul and lay hands on him so that Saul could see. Ananias' response, "*Lord, I have heard from many about this man, how much harm he did to Thy saints at Jerusalem; and here he has authority from the chief priests to bind all who call upon Thy name*" (Acts 9:13-14 NASB). God then tells Ananias, "*Go, for he is a chosen instrument of Mine, to bear My name before the Gentiles and kings and the sons of Israel*" (Acts 9:15 NASB).

Fiona said that she prayed she would act like Ananias, who was faithful when fearful. Our role in evangelism boils down to our obedience to God. The Holy Spirit is the one who does a mighty work in peoples' hearts. Soon after that we met neighbors from Afghanistan, the Ivory Coast, Albania, and many more war-torn nations. As Fiona said,

"Who knows what God will do?" Right before our eyes, He may transform the heart and life of another Saul. We can obediently share the good news about Jesus Christ today.

Has God challenged you to get outside your comfort zone during your practice of evangelism? Ananias had Saul; to whom has God led you to reach out?

____

____

The Great Commission

Then Jesus came to them and said, "All authority in heaven and on earth has been given to me. Therefore go and make disciples of all nations, baptizing them in the name of the Father and of the Son and of the Holy Spirit, and teaching them to obey everything I have commanded you. And surely I am with you always to the very end of the age" (Matt 28:18-20).

*So when they met together, they asked him, "Lord, are you at this time going to restore the kingdom to Israel?" He said to them: "It is not for you to know the times or dates the Father has set by his own authority. But you will receive power when the Holy Spirit comes on you; and you will be my witnesses in Jerusalem, and in all Judea and Samaria, and to the ends of the earth" (*Acts 1:6-8).

In both of these passages, Jesus taught His followers about missions. Here's what he taught:
1) God instructs all of us to play a role. (We can pray, go, and give financially.)
2) God wants every nation to hear His gospel.
3) God has ultimate authority. Believers through the power of the Holy Spirit can serve as faithful ambassadors at home and around the world.
4) God promises His presence.

This year think of a missions goal for yourself. If you have not already served in local, state, national, or international missions projects, speak with your minister this week.

Take time today to study Scripture, meditate on God's Word, and apply the lesson to your life. Please read Acts 9:1-19. Write down your personal missions goal for the next 12 months.

____

____

____

Day 4 Health Bite

Perhaps you are more motivated to maintain your workout program if others encourage you. If so, many resources are available to you. In your area will be health clubs, recreation centers, YMCA's, running and bicycle stores, and community colleges. They will offer a variety of services, such as group classes, weight machines, and personal trainers. Also many websites can assist you in developing your exercise program; many sites are full of fitness information.

So do whatever is necessary to get started on your personal fitness regime and the faithfulness required to continue it through your lifetime. Begin it now. However, here's a gentle word of warning. In any long-term fitness program can be setbacks and injuries. Injuries can result from a variety of circumstances such as sprained ankles, muscle pulls, and tendonitis, to name a few. I know the pain and psychological trauma that they inflict on the active person. Through these injuries I have found that the best solution is to find a substitute activity. A stationary bike or treadmill walking can be a viable alternative. Care for the injury so that you will be able to participate soon with renewed motivation. Once you quit, inactivity becomes a habit.

God is always working in our lives, so don't give up. "*Strength! Courage! Don't be timid; don't get discouraged. God, your God, is with you every step you take*" (Josh. 1:9 The Message).

Not only will you look and feel better, you will be better able to serve the Lord, our God!

Challenge: Walk 55 minutes.
Do 12 push-ups.
Do 35 crunches.

Week 6 - Day 5

Wrapping It Up

Memory Verse:

Then Jesus came to them and said, "All authority in heaven and on earth has been given to me. Therefore go and make disciples of all nations, baptizing them in the name of the Father and of the Son and of the Holy Spirit, and teaching them to obey everything I have commanded you. And surely I am with you always, to the very end of the age" (Matt. 28:18-20).

At the end of a Bible study, mission trip, or program, how do you determine success? Specifically, how do you evaluate the spiritual growth or development of yourself or others?

Today at the end of our study of evangelism and this course, please turn to and read Luke 10:1-24.

We will begin our study in verse 17. This passage provides an example of an eventful mission project and how Jesus tells those involved in the project to define *success.*

Evangelism: a spiritual battle

Please write down the words of imagery that Jesus uses to describe the spiritual victory the disciples describe as they debrief from their journey.

___

___

___

Here we find the disciples' excitement over transformed lives. On this mission trip, the Lord has given them the power to drive out demons and heal the sick—the power to continue the work without fear of harm. Imagine the success! The excitement!

One key aspect in this passage is the emphasis on the spiritual battle won. Going out to share the good news about Jesus, the practice of evangelism means that you enter a spiritual war zone.

He told them, "The harvest is plentiful, but the workers are few. Ask the Lord of the harvest, therefore, to send out workers into his harvest field. Go! I am sending you out like lambs among wolves" (Luke 10:2-3).

When He dies and rises again in three days, Jesus Christ ultimately seals His victory over Satan. But the spiritual battles here are only smaller victories in preparation of Jesus' ultimate sacrifice. These disciples specifically prepare the fields of harvest for the coming of the Messiah.

The disciples take seriously their jobs; their message remains the same despite people's acceptance. We have much the same challenge—to prepare the way of the Messiah, Who will return again. We share the gospel regardless of how popular the message appears.

We as Christ-followers have been called out to share God's good news with the entire world. When you work in the field and share the gospel, you will find spiritual victories in individual lives. Some turn from addictions, idols, or false teaching to the one true God.

We have reason for excitement! This calls for rejoicing among believers. We can claim a victory. Yet, in the middle of debriefing and celebrating, Jesus reminds them of their source of greatest joy.

What does He say?

____

____

Superior transformation

The most significant transformation we find is in salvation—the freeing of a person enslaved by sin. This one event is placed high up on a pedestal as the most important day in a life. All other life events, recommitments, and continued transformations fall behind salvation in importance. Why do we consider salvation our greatest cause for joy?

In Luke 10 we find the twofold answer. First, our eternal residence is fixed in heaven with God. At the beginning of this study I mentioned the spiritual and physical journeys each of us travels. Yet, we have a specific destination. We journey home. This life provides many opportunities to surrender to and serve God. We have the ability and responsibility to give God our best in all aspects of life. But without an ultimate goal—the reward of heaven—the practice of spiritual disciples remains meaningless. Why share the good news? We have God's guarantee that He went to prepare a place for all believers and the He will return soon.

Second, our salvation represents the greatest transformation possible. When Jesus died and rose again, He offered us a complete cleansing of our sin and the ability to live a new way of life when we obey Him.

At the point of salvation, we find the beginning of our journey. On this earth we journey focused on home. Along the road we will see transformation in our lives and others that occurs only through the power of God. In all we can count as a success a life of surrender and obedient service.

Today please read and meditate on John 14:1-6. Take time to celebrate your salvation. Recommit your life to follow Christ.

Day 5 Health Bite

Congratulations! You have reached the conclusion of this six-week journey toward better health and wellness. Take time to evaluate your progress!

Go back to the very first question that you were asked at week 1. On a scale of 1 to 10 (1=poor, 10=excellent) how do you view your current "health"? _____

Has it changed during the time you've been involved in this study? If so, how?

____

____

____

During the last few weeks what change or concept has significantly impacted your health?

____

____

Do you desire to continue healthy habits? Why or why not?

____

____

Describe how you would you like to see your health different six months from now.

____

____

Here are strategies that will help keep you focused on continuing your journey to good health. We'll call them the **five P's to Success.**
1. Pre-plan: Plan meals ahead so you are more in control of your food choices and meal timing.
2. Pre-plate: This will help limit "mindless" grazing!
3. Portion size: Keep your plate "colorful"; limit calorie-dense foods. Try applying the Plate Method (page 46) at least 85 percent of the time.
4. Pleasure: A variety of flavorful foods will help keep you interested in healthy meals. Let your creativity go wild in the kitchen!
5. Partner with someone: Share the struggles and successes with a person who can encourage and support you.

I pray each of you will reach your ultimate vision for wellness and that you will seek the Lord in this endeavor! I hope this health section has impacted your life in a positive way and that it will better equip you to serve the Lord. Remember that your journey toward wellness is a journey that is ongoing while we are here on Earth but complete when we reach Perfection in Eternity!

Sources

Week 1, Day 1

1. James Strong, *The Strongest Strong's: Exhaustive Concordance of the Bible*, eds. John R. Kohlenberger III and James A. Swanson, 21st ed. (Grand Rapids: Zondervan, 2001), 1615, 1637.

2. B.B. Warfield, "Inspiration", in *International Standard Bible Encyclopedia*, ed. G. Bromiley (Grand Rapids: Eerdmans, 1988), 840.

Week 1, Day 2

1. D.A. Carson, *New Bible Commentary: 21st Century Edition,* 4th ed., Leicester, England. (Downers Grove, IL: Inter-Varsity Press, 1994), S. Ps. 33:20-34:19.

Week 1, Day 3

1. Strong, 1607.

2. Ibid., 1265, 1573.

Week 1, Day 4

1. C.S. Lewis, *The Weight of Glory: And Other Addresses* (San Francisco: HarperSanFrancisco and HarperCollins, 1976, c. 1949, revised 1980P, 153, 4.

2. Strong, 1576.

3. Ibid., 1581.

Week 1, Day 5

1. Larry Richards, *The Bible Reader's Companion,* vol. S (Wheaton, IL: Victor Books, 1991), S. 2:756.

2. Warren W. Wiersbe, *The Bible Exposition Commentary* (Wheaton, IL: Victor Books, 1996, c1989, S. 2 Titus 3:1).

3. Kenneth L. Barker and others, eds., *Zondervan NIV Study Bible: Fully Revised* (Grand rapids: Zondervan, 1985, 1995, 2002), 1885.

4. Richards, S. 843.

Week 2, Day 2

1. John F. Walvoord and Roy B. Zuck, *The Bible Knowledge Commentary: An Exposition of Scriptures* (Wheaton, IL: Victor Books, 1983c-1985).

Week 2, Day 3

1. "Idaho Plate Method", *www.platemethod.com.* Also referenced in Rizor H., Smith M., Thomas K., Harker J., Rich M., "Practical Nutrition: The Idaho Plate Method", *Practical Diebetology,* 1988: 17:42-45.

2. Richard J. Foster, *Celebration of Discipline: The Path to Spiritual Growth,* 25th Anniversary ed. (San Francisco: HarperSanFrancisco, HarperCollins, 1998m 1988, c. 1978), 33.

Week 2, Day 4

1. Walvoord and Zuck, S. 2:62.

2. Richards, S. 620.

Week 2, Day 5

1. Strong, 1802.

Week 3, Day 1

1. A.W. Tozer, *Whatever Happened to Worship?* ed, Gerald B. Smith (Camp Hill, PA: Christian, 1985), 78.

2. Tozer, *The Knowledge of the Holy: The Attributes of God: Their Meaning in the Christian Life* (San Francisco: HarperSanFrancisco, HarperCollins, 1961), vii-viii.

Week 3, Day 2

1. Louie Giglio, *The Air I Breathe: Worship as a Way of Life* (Sisters, OR: Multnomah, 2003), 9.

2. *The New Merriam-Webster Dictionary*, ed. Frederick C. Mish (Springfield: MA: Merriam-Webster, 1989), 353.

Week 3, Day 4

1. Foster, 190-192.

2. Walvoord and Zuck, S. 1:1045.

3. William J. Reynolds, ed., *Baptist Hymnal,* 1975 ed. (Nashville, TN: Convention Press, 1975), 111.

Week 3, Day 5

1. Foster, 190-192.

Week 4, Day 4

1. Strong, 860.

Week 4, Day 5

1. Walvoord and Zuck, S. 2:532.

Week 5, Day 2

1. Dallas Willard, *The Spirit of the Disciplines: Understanding How God Changes Lives.* San Francisco: HarperSanFrancisco, HarperCollins, 1988.

Week 5, Day 3

1. Walvoord and Zuck, S. 1:1538.

2. Richards, S. 572.

3. Ibid.

4. Walvoord and Zuck.

5. Strong, 1556.

6. Walvoord and Zuck.

Week 5, Day 4

1. Walvoord and Zuck, S: 1:1541.

2. Ibid.

Week 6, Day 1

1. Walvoord and Zuck, S. 2:244.

Week 6, Day 2

1. *www.wycliff.org* (accessed Jan. 9, 2008)

Leader Guide

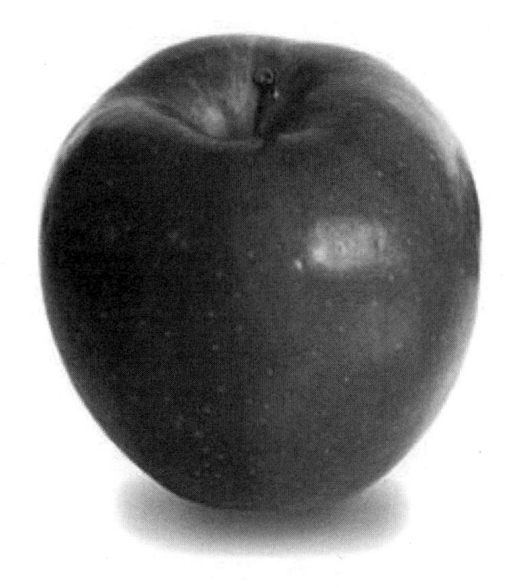

Leader Guide

Fit to Serve is a comprehensive, six-week Bible study on spiritual disciplines, nutrition, and exercise. This interdisciplinary study promotes the spiritual and physical health of Christ-followers.

Leader qualifications

You meet the criteria to lead a *Fit to Serve* Bible-study group if you have these three qualifications. First, **be a Christ-follower** (Rom. 3:23; 6:23; 10:9-10). Confess that every person has messed up—sinned, that they deserve punishment, and that they need a Savior. Believe that Jesus Christ was sent to earth as fully God and fully man to pay for the sins of the world and that Jesus Christ died and three days later rose again. Based on His victory over sin and death, He offers salvation, which you accept. Second, **seek to follow Jesus, your Lord** (John 3:16-21; Eph. 4:1-5:21). Besides believing, you regularly seek to obey God with every aspect of your life. Does this mean you never sin? No. But it means you genuinely try to obey God. Third, you **willingly take on the task of leading a small group** as a way to serve God and build up the church of Jesus Christ (Rom. 12:3-8). This involves additional responsibility. We encourage you to pray daily for your group members, seek to get to know each person who attends this Bible study, and serve the team. Include all of the members in discussion. Encourage them along their spiritual and physical journeys.

Setting up a group

1. Pray. Again and again Scripture tells us to pray. In fact, prayer is one of the spiritual disciplines we will study. So start now and keep it up.
2. Identify a core group. Determine who will attend the study. Do you plan to offer the curriculum with an existing Bible-study group or gather a small group of friends for the study? After identifying a group, you then can plan for the group's needs. For example, do you need to arrange for child care?
3. Find an appropriate time and place. If you hope to lead this study at your church, plan a time to meet with the minister over discipleship groups or with whatever staff person you deem appropriate and propose the idea of a *Fit to Serve* Bible study at your church. Please respect the staff member's suggestions about the schedule and place to meet. Determine how much time you need to conduct the group. We suggest you allow at least one hour to conduct the group.
4. Plan for and publicize the study. Depending on your core group and after gaining approval from church leaders, if necessary, start getting the word out. You could post signs around the church and send out invitations through emails, blogs, phone calls, or

the ever-successful method—word of mouth.
5. Order books. Plan to order the books at least six weeks in advance. You can order this Bible study at *www.hannibalbooks.com* or call 1-800-747-0738.
6. Plan the room arrangement.
7. Pray again. 1 Thessalonians 5:17

Preparation for the class

• Pray for each group member and for all specified prayer requests.
• Pray for God's truth to be taught and for each individual as he or she seeks to apply the spiritual disciplines and health changes.
• Prepare for the class discussion.
• Make sure the room has the necessary items: chairs, pens/pencils, projector, laptop, and screen.
• Complete the weekly homework.
• Prepare a sign-in sheet, nametags, and pens.
• As leader at all times try to stay at least one week ahead of the group members as you complete your weekly work so you are prepared with any questions that might arise among group members.

Group times

• Spend the first few minutes mingling with the class. Make sure you welcome each person by name.
• Begin with prayer. Take class prayer requests. If the class is small, ask for the requests and pray. If the class is large, provide either prayer cards or a prayer list for members to share specific requests. Identify the confidentiality level of each request. If applicable email the list to all members during the week or assign the task to another person.
• As a group read the Scripture memory verse out loud. Repeat the previous week's verse to help the class remember.
• A class lesson guide follows this leader introductory material. Read the class lesson guide thoroughly before each group meeting. As leader prepare to present this material to your class. You will find a guide for both the Bible study portion and the health focus. You do not have to present this material word for word and commit it to rote memory, but do become familiar enough with the material so that you do not have to read it. Prepare yourself so you can readily explain the content to group members while you make eye-contact with them. Prepare to lead them in the discussion time. Be familiar enough with the material that you have a general idea how members are to properly answer questions asked.

Wrapping up

> *Two are better than one, because they have a good return for their work: If one falls down, his friend can help him up. But pity the man who falls and has no one to help him up!* (Eccl. 4:9-10).

God designed church members to play unique roles but also to work together in unity. Working together allows us to accomplish more. One way we can do this is by separating a group into small groups (four or fewer) or accountability groups (two people). Preferably separate genders unless you choose to establish a group of married couples. Then as you progress through the study and set and apply goals, the members can pray for and provide individual encouragement for each other. During the first group time, ask the class members to divide into accountability or small groups.

Wrapping up class

1. Encourage class members to complete the homework assignments and to memorize the Scripture-memory verse for the next week.
2. Allow a period of breakout time (suggested time: 10-15 minutes) for small groups or accountability groups. Within each group ask members to share the progress about their health goals and lessons or experiences from practicing the spiritual disciplines. Encourage the small groups to close in prayer and quietly leave once members finish their discussion and prayer time.
3. As leader, start and end the class on time. Child-care providers may be waiting for members to pick up their children. Worship services and other church activities may start immediately after class time, so please avoid detaining persons in your class from participating in the activities that follow your group meeting. Be reliable in your group-management skills.

Class Lesson Week 1

Leader presentation

(The leader presents the following lesson on the spiritual discipline of studying Scripture.)

Today we will start the class discussion in Deuteronomy 32. Please ask members to read Deuteronomy 32:47a.

Moses speaks these words to the Israelites as they embark on a new chapter. He has given the people the law of the Lord. They prepare to enter Canaan, the Promised Land.

Forty years earlier the Israelites have embarked on the same Mount. At that time they prepare for their entry of the land by sending out 12 spies from each of the tribes to scout out the land; all but two return with a discouraging reports (Num. 13).

God disciplines the Israelites for their lack of faith by sending them to wander in the wilderness until the disobedient generation dies (Num. 14). In Deuteronomy 32 the next generation of Israelites with the few faithful leaders—Moses, Joshua, and Caleb—face the Promised Land again.

Moses sings to his people about God's faithfulness and their history of disobedience (Deut. 32). In this pivotal moment, Moses encourages them to believe in their God, to obey the Law, and to keep their covenant with Him.

Moses knows the Israelites' entry into the Promised Land will bring challenges. He charges them to stay close to their God. They can do this by recognizing the importance of God's law in their daily lives and by obeying His commandments.

What does the future hold? When they face new challenges in the land, will they believe God and obediently follow His commands? Will they listen to and obey the words of the great "I AM" who leads their people safely out of Egypt?

Moses personally knows the consequences of disobedience. He, too, has acted unfaithfully to the Lord by overstepping God's instructions and hitting a rock to provide water for the Israelites (Num. 20). As a consequence he will not enter the Promised Land.

The Israelites long to enter the Promised Land—a land of rest and plenty, a land in which wandering will cease. Moses prepares his people: he cautions them, tells them about their God's character, reminds them of their ancestors' mistakes, and encourages them to live according to God's Words—the relevant and powerful Words of God.

Questions for the group:

Ask members to discuss the following questions:

• How do you view Scripture?

• What relationship do you see between one's perspective of Scripture and his or her willingness to apply its teachings personally?

• Compare and contrast the difference between the Israelites who do not think they can take the land versus the outlook of Moses, Joshua, and Caleb.

• Rhetorical question: Which group do you tend to act like?

The Israelites have excellent leaders such as Moses, Joshua, and Caleb. For example Caleb does not hesitate to follow the Lord personally and to encourage others to do the same (Num. 13:30 and 14:24).

• Do you have a friend or family member who encouraged you to study and obey God's Word? If so, who?

• How did the person encourage you? What difference did this encouragement make?

Scripture is truth—an active and applicable word for your life. Moses encourages the Israelites to obey. This is a call for obedience to us, too.

Encouragement to recommit

Now please turn to Joshua 22:1-5 and read this passage. Moses dies just before the Israelites enter the Promised Land; Joshua takes over as their leader. In Joshua 22 we find the Israelites living in Canaan. They have taken over much of the land God has given to them.

Again we find ourselves reading a passage that marks the end of a great leader's service. This time Joshua admonishes the Israelites to obey God's commandments.

• Have you ever had a time–a new life stage—in which you noticed a need to recommit your life to the Lord? Recommitment can occur after a time of faithful obedience.

In this chapter Joshua encourages the Israelites to remain faithful to God even after a time of victory and peace. In Joshua 22:5 He specifically gives them five words of advice. Below I have listed them.

1. Love the Lord your God.
2. Walk in all His ways.
3. Obey His commands.
4. Hold fast to Him.
5. Serve Him with all your heart and all your soul.

Ask members to discuss the following questions:

- **Discuss the role that each of these tips plays in your study of Scripture and obedience to God.**

- **Ask members to give a couple of life examples for each tip. (For example, you show your love for God by prioritizing your time with Him—the time you spend alone reading Scripture and praying.) Try to let one example relate to the spiritual discipline of studying Scripture, but you can expand the ideas beyond this topic.**

(The leader then presents the following health and fitness lesson to the group.)

The Bible tells us Scripture is *God-breathed and useful for teaching, rebuking, correcting, and training in righteousness, so that the man of God may be thoroughly equipped for every good work* (2 Tim. 3:16). The words of the Bible represent God's roadmap for our lives. I'm always amazed at how the stories, parables, and Christ's teachings relate so relevantly to life now in the 21st century. One vivid memory from my high-school years illustrates how Scripture tremendously impacted my life as it challenged me to discontinue unhealthy habits!

Early in my high-school years I was very active in sports and dance, but I would not consider myself petite like many of my friends were. I was considered more "big-boned". In my junior year, I decided to get "into shape", so I began by running around our family garden in Pennsylvania. This quickly turned from my barely being able to run a mile to running avidly and joining a local gym—both healthy things for a young woman of 16 until they were taken too far. The positive comments and praise of how good I looked turned me into a workout junkie and a selective eater. The Lord decided to give me a "wake-up" call when I looked at pictures from our family beach vacation that next summer. They revealed a very thin and unhealthy person. That evoked a deep sense of fear in me; thankfully this put a stop to my weight loss. God used pictures and the words of 1 Corinthians 6:19: *Do you now know that your body is a temple of the Holy Spirit, who is in you, whom you have received from God?* to allow me to see that I was not taking care of the body He had entrusted to me. I was abusing it; that was a turning point toward a life of better health, a commitment to a body for Christ, and a career path to become a dietitian.

Do you believe you "honor the Lord" with the food you eat and the way to choose to care for the precious gift that God has given you—your body? During the next six weeks I challenge you to wrestle with this question. What does this look like for you personally? Each of us has a unique shape and frame that was specifically created just for us; some are "petite" and some "big-boned". Some struggle desperately with losing weight; some struggle desperately with how they use (or abuse) food. Regardless of your struggle, my passion for each of you is that you would learn how to use food to "honor" the Lord. This does not only mean achieving a healthy weight but also achieving a healthy relationship with food. Both your body and the nourishment provided in the form of food are gifts from above. How we use them is a choice our Father extends to each of us.

Group discussion

As leader, ask members to state what the word *wellness* means to them. Does it imply the absence of disease, successfully controlling disease, or making the cover of *SHAPE* or *Muscle and Fitness* magazine? *Wellness* is a term we use very loosely in our culture. Webster's defines *wellness* as "the condition of being healthy or sound, especially as the result of proper diet and exercise". Overall wellness can include physical, emotional, financial, and spiritual health. Achieving good health in these areas does not occur without great effort. Wellness also can be viewed as "an active process of becoming aware of and making choices toward a more successful existence."

Questions for the group

Ask members to discuss the following questions:

- **How do you define optimal health and wellness?**

- **How do you think God would have us honor Him through our eating habits?**

- **How does our "culture" affect our view of health and weight?**

- **Is the bathroom scale a good means to use to measure "success" when our "health" is concerned?**

- **Use the Body Mass Index Chart in the appendix o calculate your BMI, which is associated with risk of disease based on weight. What circumstances may make this means less than reliable?**

Individually this week

Ask members to thoughtfully and prayerfully consider these three questions. They may write their answers in the blanks provided.

Do my current lifestyle habits, including what I choose to eat, honor the Lord and nourish the body He has entrusted to me? Why or why not?

____

____

Where does pursuing healthy eating and exercise habits fall on my "priority list" of life?

____

____

What is my "ultimate vision" of good health?

____

____

What two to three things could I make a focus this week to improve my health?

____

____

Class Lesson Week 2

Leader presentation

(The leader presents the following lesson on the spiritual discipline of prayer.)

This week we begin our study on the spiritual discipline of prayer. Prayer is direct communication with God. In various passages the Bible instructs Christ-followers on how to pray. During the homework this week we will break down one such passage: the Lord's Prayer (Matt. 6). Today let us turn to Philippians 4:4–7. These four verses help us focus on the role of the discipline of prayer in our spiritual journey.

A greeting

In Philippians 4:4 the Bible says, "*Rejoice in the Lord always. I will say it again: Rejoice!*" Daily in passing conversation I offer the salutation, "Hope you have a great day." Why do this? It serves as a reminder for myself and others—we have a choice. Decide to rejoice in all circumstances. In much the same way Paul encourages the readers of his letter.

A motivation

In Philippians 4:5 Paul gives an instruction to rejoice when he says, *Let your gentleness be evident to all. The Lord is near.* What gives Paul the right to state this exhortation? Well, he lives it. In his letter to the Philippians and in other epistles we find that Paul rejoices when he receives beatings, imprisonments, and faces hunger. From his own personal example, we recognize that rejoicing results from a decision as opposed to external circumstances or internal emotions.

Set a goal

For the rest of our lives we travel a spiritual and physical journey. As motivation for our obedience, we focus our sights on heaven—our home. *The Lord is near,* says Philippians 4:5b. Well-respected theologians have taken this verse a couple of ways: 1) that God's presence is close by us, and 2) that Jesus' second coming is near or close at hand. Based on my personal study I am inclined to think *near* refers to Christ's second coming. I think this verse encourages us to live with intention. The choice to rejoice and the decision to live with patience emerges from an eternal perspective.

Put in a request

When you face a struggle, have you ever mentally told yourself not to fret but felt your impending stress level and possibly even your blood pressure rising. What now? Have you shown yourself incapable of acting on Paul's exhortation? On your own, yes.

In Philippians 4:6 the Bible says, *Do not be anxious about anything, but in everything, by prayer and petition, with thanksgiving, present your requests to God.*" Here we find the introduction to prayer. Prayer involves placing a request—calling out to God for help. In the Lord's Prayer this week we will see this point expanded on. A professor pointed out for me that prayer consists of various requests. Look at Scripture each aspect or guideline on prayer ultimately boils down to asking God for something.

Paul encourages us to pray. Pray about everything, he says. Petition the Lord.

How do you begin to practice the spiritual discipline of prayer? As Paul encourages us, pray about what is going on now—both the good and the bad. Place them at the feet of your Savior—a Savior that you know will return again—a victorious King you can trust.

The end result

When you return home after a challenging day, how do you feel? Stressed out? Why? We need peace in a world that lacks it.

Pray, Paul exhorts us. In Philippians 4:7 he writes, *And the peace of God, which transcends all understanding, will guard your hearts and your minds in Christ Jesus.* Philippians 4:7. He tells us that the peace of God—peace that lasts—a peace the world cannot offer—will enter your life. A peace beyond our intellectual understanding will descend on you. It is a peace that protects your mind and your heart. This peace originates from your Savior. This peace occurs as you seek God through the spiritual discipline of prayer.

Discussion questions

Ask members to discuss the following questions:

• How often do you practice the spiritual discipline of prayer?

• How do you cope with stress?

• What do you find is a common source of stress? Note: Many turn to food as a way to cope with stress. This week ask God to help you address your struggles at the root, instead of seeking temporary comfort with food. Take time and present your requests to God.

• Will you commit to regularly turn this issue to the Lord in prayer? You don't have to kneel down or close your eyes. But when you find yourself faced with this challenge again, immediately seek the Lord in prayer.

(The leader then presents to the group the following health and fitness lesson.)

In both the Old and New Testaments the Lord provides food for his people when they are in need. He feeds the crowd of 5,000 with fish and bread, provides quail and manna for the Israelites, and gives locust and honey to John in the desert. We live in a land of "plenty" and "excess" in which we easily can abuse this luxury through overindulgence. Read Exodus 16. How does the Lord teach the Israelites to trust Him to provide for their basic needs on a daily basis? What happens if they take too much manna and keep it until morning? Reflect on these three examples mentioned above. What type of food is provided? When and how much food does God choose to give? How is it received?

In the case of the Israelites, the Lord knows they need food in the morning and at night. He creates us to eat regularly throughout the day for energy and nourishment. Our metabolism is what turns fuel (food) into energy. So for optimal energy and weight control, the act of eating helps to keep our metabolism fired up!

Interestingly these examples of God's provision demonstrate the importance of having both protein (fish, quail, locust) and carbohydrate (bread, manna, honey) to meet our body's requirements. Carbohydrates are easily and quickly broken down into glucose and used by the body for energy (we store carbohydrate calories only when we overindulge). Notice how much the Lord provides in each example—just enough for each person to be satisfied. Protein is necessary to maintain lean muscle mass and healthy immune systems. More work is required for our bodies to break this down, thus making us feel full longer. If God provides only carbohydrates in these examples, the people may continue to feel hungry. If only protein is provided, then energy level will be diminished; they may be unable to complete the task the Lord had given them. The people offer thanksgiving and praise for the provision of food. Are we in the habit of doing this today?

Often we may fail to balance our macronutrients throughout the day to provide optimal energy. (Macronutrients are carbohydrates, protein, and fat sources.) For example, a piece of fruit is a very healthy snack in the afternoon. However, because it is a carbohydrate, it may keep you satisfied for only a short while. Pair the fruit with a protein source such as low-fat cheese. You may feel a bit more satisfied and less hungry by dinner! Fiber-rich foods such as whole grains also are great for keeping us full longer. This week, try to use the model on the next page to balance your plate at meal times. Also, find ways to thank the Lord for the provision of food and fluids this week. How might this mindful act of thanks have an impact on how you view and approach the food you are about to enjoy?

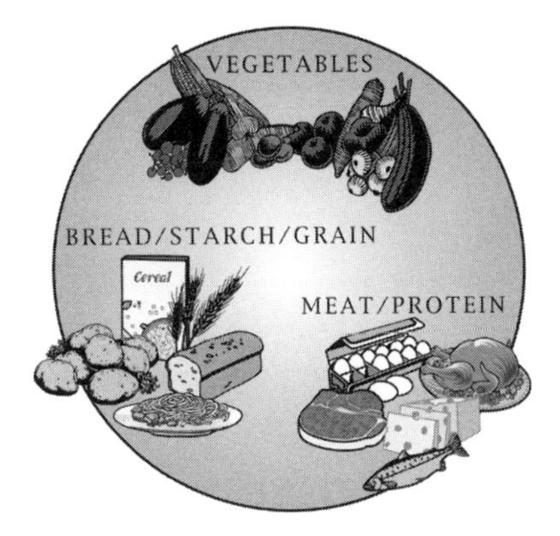

Questions for the group

Ask members to discuss the following questions:

- What types of food choices do you select when you are over-hungry? How would your choices differ if you were mild-to-moderately hungry?

- Does planning meals ahead of time have an impact on the type of food choices or volume of food eaten?

- Compare your last meal with the "Plate Method" (above). How is your "balance"?

- Evaluate how your energy level may be affected by the food choices you make.

Individually this week

Ask members to thoughtfully and prayerfully consider these three questions. They may write their answers in the blanks provided.

Consider setting three to five goals you believe you can achieve this week. Below are some examples.

- I will limit/ include protein portion to 3 to 4 ounces at meal times (lunch/dinner) ____ days this week.

- I will use the "Plate Method" concept at least ______ times this week.

- I will thank the Lord for creating food and be mindful to choose food that nourishes my body at least ______ days this week.

- I will choose more "whole foods" this week by ________________________.

- On ________________ I will pre-plan my meals for the week.

Class Lesson Week 3

Leader presentation

(The leader presents the following lesson on the spiritual discipline of worship.)

This week we begin our study of the spiritual discipline of worship. During this class time we will look at the Christ-follower's role in worship. Let's start by reading Romans 12:1:*Therefore, I urge you, brothers, in view of God's mercy, to offer your bodies as living sacrifices, holy and pleasing to God—this is your spiritual act of worship.*

According to this verse, worship flows into every aspect of life. A correct view of God impacts the purpose of our work, our attitudes, and how we respond to others.

Let's take a moment as a class and discuss how we literally practice the spiritual discipline of worship seven days a week.

Let me share with you this parable.

Three to Four Hours a Day

A theologian was sent to a small town by the sea. His home was filled with books; it resembled a library. Each morning he studied diligently to gain knowledge; in the evenings he taught the educated folk in town, for a small fee, of course. They liked to hear his lofty monologues. Each day after dinner the neighbor's boy would listen by the fence to hear this brilliant theologian. After the theologian ended the class, the young lad would run to the gate and ask questions about the lecture. This man found the young boy's questions annoying and so dismissed him. "I haven't the time to talk with you, lad. I have journals to read and books to write. Plus I only get three to four hours of sleep each night. I really don't have time for you, little boy . . . go and run along home."

A flood lambasted a neighboring town. The theologian thought God wanted him to join the rebuilding effort. So he made a step of faith and left his books to provide spiritual support for those in need. He always went out with disaster relief teams. No danger scared him off. For several months he slept on hard gym floors and tolerated cold showers. One evening he had enough of the rough living conditions; his dinner was particularly poor, so he went to complain to the chef. On entering the kitchen, he found a young man stirring a pot of beef stew.

"This stew is pitiful," the theologian complained, "I would rather have grits."

The young man looked up from the 32-gallon pot and recognized the theologian. "You are my neighbor!" he almost shouted. The tired lad grinned from ear to ear. "Tell me what you have seen."

The theologian stood silent. He recognized the young man as his annoying and inquisitive neighbor. "It is a natural disaster. The workers would do better with satisfied stomachs. Just keep on cooking." With that, the theologian quickly turned to go.

The man ran after him. "Would you like coffee? Can we sit and catch up?"

"Nope," the theologian replied. "I am about to leave for a rescue mission that will take at least three to four hours today. Don't have time, you see. It will take at least three to four hours."

After years traveling the world and serving in disaster relief, the theologian retired. He returned home expecting to see friends, family, and his adoring students from years past. Instead he returned to an empty house filled with books. For a man in his 90's, he got along fine. He had a microwave, food, ESPN, and a reclining chair that doubled as a bed for those late-night NCAA championships. He didn't have to miss a thing. Then on Thanksgiving, he felt lonely. That afternoon he heard a knock on his door. He stretched his sore bones enough to shuffle to the entryway and saw a grown man on his front porch. "What do you want?" the theologian asked through the door.

The man identified himself as the neighbor's boy who returned home for Thanksgiving. "Would you like to join us for our Thanksgiving meal?" the man asked.

This time the theologian offered no excuse. "Yes . . . I can come right now."

So the neighbor's boy helped the old man cross the driveway. They entered his childhood home—a home into which the old man had never stepped foot. Over dinner the neighbors asked about the books the old man had studied and the restoration efforts in which he served. For hours they listened as he told about his sacrificial life.

As the evening began to close, the neighbor's boy walked this old man back home. Before the old man closed the door, the young man asked. "If you were to sum up your life in a statement, what would you say?"

The man held his head high, "I am a Christian. I am a good Christian. I am a Christian seven days a week, three to four hours a day."

Questions for the group

Immediately after you read the parable, ask one class member to read out loud Romans 12:1, 9-12. Next have another class member read to the class 1 Corinthians 13:1-3.

Based on the reading ask the group to discuss the following questions:

- **What does living a sacrificial life of worship mean?**

- **Did the old man in the parable practice the spiritual discipline of worship? Why or why not?**

- **Please list attitudes and actions that characterize a Christ-follower who lives a life of worship based on Romans 12 and 1 Corinthians 13.**

• As a group write a summary statement describing how a Christian can strive to worship God on a daily basis.

(The leader then presents to the group the following health and fitness lesson.)

Close your eyes for just a moment and reflect on the emotions associated with the last time you gazed on an array of color painted in the sky. Sunsets and rainbows fascinate most of us, as they evoke a sense of awe and wonder. I love rainbows. Longing to uncover the magical pot of gold at the end of the rainbow, which I did as a child, turned to something much deeper as I grew to fully understand the significance of God's handiwork.

I will never forget the summer of 1995 when my friend Robyn and I were traveling back to Pennsylvania from Georgia. I was exhausted from driving; she had cried a river of tears because of a recent broken heart. The weather was rainy and dismal, it matched both our moods. Suddenly, as if in a movie, the clouds broke away and revealed four glorious rainbows in all different directions. The impact this had on the mood in that car and on our spirits was comical. Frowns and tears, exhaustion and frustration vanished in a split-second as it turned to joy, awe, and excitement. We quickly pulled off the road and began frantically jumping up and down, taking pictures, and pointing to the awesome site around us. That day not just overwhelming beauty moved me; I also was touched by the reminder of the love and power of our Maker and His promises.

God's amazing design of vivid colors is found not only in rainbows but also in so many other areas in nature, particularly food! The amazing array of fruits and vegetables God has created deserves our attention and our admiration from childhood to adulthood. Take a few minutes this week to open your refrigerator and freezer; what "colors" do you purchase? Take inventory. Do you see more man-made "colors" than the uniquely designed fruits and vegetables God ingeniously created? Next, think about your last meal; did you have color on your plate? You may be surprised to find that "color" on your plate may brighten your mood and serve as a positive reminder of His promises to lovingly care and protect you. How could you include more of God's colorful creation in your meals and snacks this week as an act of worship and praise?

Questions for the group

Ask members to discuss the following questions:

• Discuss how taking time and acknowledging the Lord's handiwork might cause you to appreciate eating more fruit and vegetables.

• Do you have a "priority" to obtain the recommended servings of fruit and vegetables per day? Why or why not?

• Discuss the recommendation and reason for these guidelines.

• How can you fill your plate with three or more "colors" at mealtimes? Would this be something to introduce to your children or family?

• Discuss favorite fruits and vegetables. Share recipes and creative ideas to include these in your meals.

Individually this week

Ask members to thoughtfully and prayerfully consider these three questions. They may write their answers in the blanks provided.

• Do an "inventory" of your refrigerator, freezer, and pantry.

• Set some personal goals to increase your fruit/vegetable intake. (Ex. I will fill ___ percent of my plate with "color" at lunch and dinner ____ times this week. Choose a goal that is realistic; then build on this until at least 85 percent of the time you achieve this on a daily basis.)

• How will you take time to plan this into your week?

Class Lesson Week 4

Leader presentation

(The leader presents the following lesson on ministry and service)

The death of one girl changed the lives of a small group of sixth-graders. We lost a friend. But the realization that death looms taught us about ministry and service. This week we begin our study on the spiritual discipline of service.

Before and after our friend's death our teachers and parents talked with us about dying, life, and ministry. They helped us recognize how even in the hospital our friend could share about Christ and encourage other patients. She lived with intention.

They also kept our focus on the future—dreaming of the hope of heaven—living in the presence of God without pain or sickness. They challenged a group of kids to minister with everything we had at our disposal. We knew our life could end at any moment. Today mattered. What would we do with our time?

In sixth grade three of us girls decided to start a teen-age girls' mission group at our church. Our moms helped provide the materials and transportation. They encouraged us to start praying together weekly.

God used this time to show us that everyone regardless of age, education level, gender, lack or presence of resources, and skills played an important role in the ministry. Our moms helped us try out various forms of ministry. We visited the sick, fed the hungry, raised money for missions, learned about missionaries, and taught Bible studies. A group of awkward, middle-school girls recognized that God wanted to use us.

By high school the two other girls accepted a call to ministry. One is entering missions as a Bible translator; the other is attending seminary in preparation for children's ministry. I was the last to surrender to God's call. We all look back and recognize God taught us about the need for service and ministry. Our roles as servants were just as important at age 12 as they are now.

The New Testament contains four passages on spiritual gifts. One of these is Ephesians 4. Ask the class to stop and read Ephesians 4:1-16. Tell the class that you will focus on one verse in the passage—Ephesians 4:16, *From him the whole body, joined and held together by every supporting ligament, grows and builds itself up in love, as each part does its work.*

Questions for the group

Ask the group to discuss the following questions:

- **Who is the "him" to which Ephesians 4:16 refers?**

Tell the group to feel free to use a "church answer" here. Affirm that the "him" refers to Jesus Christ. Paul begins the epistle to the Ephesians by teaching doctrine. His teaching of doctrine includes teaching about Christ as our Savior.

This reminds us that the spiritual discipline of service frequently applies to the church. For our purposes in this study we will base service on ministry within or by the church.

• How does the church live out unity today?

Explain that Ephesians 4:16 tells us that the members of the body support each other in ministry. A unifying goal of service is to build up the church. This study strives to encourage you as you serve. This week in your lesson on exercise, Carol and Don give guidelines for determining your physical fitness and helpful tips to strengthen your physical body.

By practicing the spiritual discipline of service you strengthen the body of Christ. You help the church grow stronger so that all of us can serve better.

• What role does love play in the practicing the spiritual discipline of service?

Love unites believers. It joins all of the body parts together. This week as you study the spiritual discipline of service and learn about spiritual gifts, decide to love the church. Decide to love when doing so is easy and when it is challenging. A correct view and love for God will bring about a love for other believers. Recommend that members read 1 John 4:7-21 on loving the church.

(The leader then presents to the group the following health and fitness lesson.)

"I don't have time." "I'm too busy." "I don't like to sweat." As physical-education teachers we hear these complaints all the time. "Why do we have to run?" "Why do I have to do sit-ups?" "Push-ups again?" The short answer to these questions is that we do these activities because our bodies need regular physical exercise to maintain a minimum level of health and fitness.

The more complete answer to the fitness question has some important factors. First, the number-one cause of death in the United States is heart disease, followed by cancer, stroke, chronic respiratory disease, and accidents. The total amount of deaths is about two million each year! That number is huge in terms of human life—about the size of a small city. With some exceptions, these preventable deaths are the result of chronic diseases that develop over a long period of time. They are caused by our lifestyles, our habits, our weight, diet, and our choices we make each day. The factors are influenced each day by the choices we make.

In the beginning

God designs people to work physically and after the Garden of Eden fiasco commands us to do so. *So God expelled them from the Garden of Eden and sent them to work the ground* (Gen. 3:23 The Message). "*You will eat the grain of the field. By the sweat of your brow you will eat your food until you return to the ground*" (Gen. 3:18-19).

But in our 21st-century world of labor-saving devices and technology, we do not work the fields or do any other form of difficult labor. Therefore, we must work out to maintain the body created for us.

Fit to serve

Not only are we God's temple (1 Cor. 3:16-17), but Jesus teaches us to serve each other in work and deed. Eat right and engage in regular exercise for the purpose of being a more vital, healthy, energetic, and useful servant of the Lord. We want to be motivated to be physically fit to glorify God in our bodies and as His servants. *For you were called to freedom, brothers and sisters; only do not use freedom as an opportunity to indulge your flesh, but through love serve one another* (Gal. 5:13 NASB).

To serve the Lord best, we must be disciplined to become physically fit. *I don't know about you, but I'm running hard for the finish line. I'm giving it everything I've got. No sloppy living for me! I'm staying alert and in top condition* (1 Cor. 9:26-27 The Message). Take a moment to think about your example to the world. What does your physical appearance say to people you meet? What destructive health habits do you have that might destroy your witness? How does your fitness level affect your ability to share your testimony?

Mary's story

Mary was a middle-aged mother of two children. She was overweight, tired, and often depressed about the mounting responsibilities at work and home. She rarely had time for herself, so a regular exercise program was not a part of her life. A friend asked Mary to meet her one morning to walk the neighborhood. Mary was glad to meet with her friend, so they decided to walk at 6 a.m. the next morning, a half-hour earlier than Mary usually rose. That one commitment changed Mary's life! Years later, she is fit and trim, excited about her life, and uses her walk time to pray, think creatively, and organize her day.

Through the ages

The human body needs activity, as evidenced through the benefits we receive in an organized and sustained exercise program. We also know that the physical body has a natural progression of decline through life. An active lifestyle and a healthy diet help to slow this process. What are you doing to slow down your own aging process?

As we age, the body loses muscle tissue and increases in body fat because of the gradual decrease in our metabolism, coupled with less activity. Aerobic exercise and strength training can sustain muscle tissue mass at a higher level and delays changes in the metabolism. What are you doing to maintain your muscle mass? What aerobic exercise are you doing? What long-term goals do you have to slow down this aging process?

Bone density peaks at about 30 years of age. Then the bones begin to weaken. The rate of bone loss exceeds the rate of replacement; the bones become less dense and fragile. Women are at greater risk because of less bone mass in their skeletons and after menopause because of a drop in estrogen production. Again, aerobic-type activities, such as walking, and strength training with weights slows done the loss of bone density. How is your exercise program designed to prevent loss of bone density?

The heart of the matter

The leading cause of death in the United States is heart disease. About one million lives are lost each year. This significant loss is alarming. The unfortunate truth is that we often cause this preventable problem with our own lifestyle, diet, and destructive habits.

Care for your own heart. Without missing a beat it must sustain you from before birth until your death. It delivers the essential oxygen and nutrients to all the cells of the body. We cannot leave something that important to chance. Be informed and active in its care. God tells us, *Let us not lose heart in doing good, for in due time we shall reap if we do not grow weary* (Gal. 6:9).

If you have not had exercise clearance from your doctor, please do so first. Then you will begin slowly, especially if you have been away from exercise for awhile. Getting into shape is a process. It is not a quick fix. Walking is a good way to start. The idea is to elevate the heart rate for a short but sustained period and then gradually extend the time and distance. Work toward 20-45 minutes, three to five times a week.

FITT

The principles of training will assist you in planning your workout program. Use the acronym FITT to help you.

- F = Frequency of Training—how often you exercise (3-5 days a week)
- I = Intensity of Training—how forcefully you exercise (measured by your target heart rate)
- T = Time—how long you exercise (20-45 minutes)
- T = Type—the type of exercise (swim, run, walk, bike, etc.)

Conclusion

Physical exercise is a part of our daily lives and has been for many years. We hope to encourage you to continue your workouts or to begin one. In 2 Thessalonians 3:13 the Lord motivates all of us when He says, *Do not grow weary in doing what is right.* As Christians we are to serve others and be all that God wants us to be. Be spiritually and physically ready for the challenge. The discipline you develop in maintaining a lifelong workout program will also enable you to be more disciplined in your prayer and Bible-study time.

So start today and see what great and mighty things God has planned for you. *No one's ever seen or heard anything like this, never so much imagined anything quite like what God has arranged for those who love him* (1 Cor. 2:9 The Message). Don't concentrate on getting ready for swimsuit season or your high-school reunion. Getting into the best shape you can be to serve the Lord our God for as long as you live. *We pray that you'll have strength to stick it out over the long haul* (Col. 1:11 The Message).

Group discussion

Ask the group to discuss the following questions:

- **What lifestyle habits contribute to poor health?**

- **What habits promote strong, healthy bodies?**

- **How can we slow down the aging process?**

- **Take a moment to assess your weekly schedule. What role does exercise play?**

- **How can you make adaptations to help achieve a more healthy, stronger life?**

- **Is being physically healthy important for a Christ-follower? If so, why?**

- **How can a Christ-follower let his or her worldview influence his or her lifestyle?**

Individually this week

Ask members to thoughtfully and prayerfully consider these three questions. They may write their answers in the blanks provided.

- **What lifestyle habits contribute to poor health?**
- **What habits promote strong, healthy bodies?**
- **How can we slow down the aging process?**
- **Take a moment to assess your weekly schedule. What role does exercise play?**
- **How can you make adaptations to help achieve a healthier, stronger life?**
- **Is it important for a Christian to be physically healthy? If so, why?**
- **How can a Christ-follower let his or her worldview influence his or her lifestyle?**

Ask members to collect food labels to bring to class at your Week 5 session.

Class Lesson Week 5

Leader presentation

(The leader presents the following lesson on simplicity.)

Have you moved recently? I am about to move for the third time since undergraduate school. Each time my move provides a time to simplify. Who wants to pack up everything, anyway? The moves let me purge from life the unnecessary. I have done away with the pastel décor from my college apartment and even my favorite Papason chair from high school. Eliminating the excess allows me to focus on the present life stage and how I can best bring glory to God. This is where we find the spiritual discipline of simplicity.

What benefits do I have from the constant simplification? I spend less time taking care of my possessions. I need less space. Best of all, my cleaning list has decreased from an entire day to just a half-day.

In much the same way as I got rid of furniture, files, and décor, the practice of simplicity allows me to assess various areas of my life to see if I need to purge other aspects that take my resources and time. The opportunity of this stage in life will not last forever. How can I bring glory to God now?

King Solomon wrote the book of Ecclesiastes and a portion of the book of Proverbs. Ecclesiastes presents his contemplations on life after pursuing its treasures. Read aloud Ecclesiastes 5:10-17.

Questions for the group

Ask members to discuss the following questions:

- **What does Solomon give us as the purpose of labor?**

Tell the group, Labor can reveal our true desires. By taking part in simplicity and solitude we are challenged to reveal what we use to motivate us. Your primary motivator will determine your willingness to practice the spiritual disciplines of simplicity.

- **How could you practice simplicity in your life now? Discuss one way you could simplify.**

Read aloud to the group Ecclesiastes 5:18-20. These verses address contentment.

- **What approach does Solomon encourage about career and possessions?**

• If you ranked yourself on the contentment scale, with 10 as the highest, what level of contentment do you have in life?

Close by telling the group, Solitude provides the time to assess your contentment and renew your commitment to follow God. Will you break from work to spend time getting to know God intimately?

(The leader then presents the following health and fitness lesson to the group.)

Are you a FOODIE? Do you enjoy going to the grocery store or farmer's market more than you do your local mall? I confess—I do! However, for many people this is a chore that leaves them frustrated and confused. Can you relate to the following scenario?

You decided to dash into the market to pick up a few items. As you whip down the snack-food aisle, you observe women and men attempting to juggle boxes and bags as they compare the food labels. They stand in the aisle for what seems like aeons. They may shake their heads, pull out their cell phones to make a call, or hastily put all products back on the shelf and stomp away to the next aisle!

If you are attempting to eat well, are you confident that the foods you are choosing are healthy? Or do you find shopping may cause anxiety, frustration, or even border on insanity! Use the following tips to become a savvy and health-smart shopper!

1. Plan ahead: Each week commit to a certain day and time to shop. Plan meals and snacks for the week. Be proactive; keep a pen and pad on the frig to note when you run out of something. This makes the next step much easier!

2. Make a list: This will help your shopping trip to be more efficient and can help minimize impulse purchases. But don't let your list prevent you from looking for and trying new healthy foods to add variety!

3. Do not go to the store hungry. Set yourself up for success and shop after you have eaten a good meal. If you are running on empty, drink water or buy a piece of fruit to munch on!

4. Shop the perimeter of the store. Fresh fruit, veggies, meats, and dairy products typically are found around the edge of the store. Try to ensure that more than half of your cart is filled with "perimeter" foods!

5. Go with a positive and healthy mindset. Make the grocery shopping experience pleasant. Avoid going when you are crunched for time or in a bad mood. This may negatively affect your food choices and lead to purchasing "comfort" foods.

6. Read the food label. Look at the food label in its entirety instead of choosing only one or two areas to compare. Use these quick guidelines to help you.

SERVING SIZE: Start first by looking at the serving size. If you eat three times the serving size, then triple the numbers on the label!

FAT: Focus on limiting saturated fat and trans fats that can lead to chronic disease. Saturated fat is found in high-fat animal sources, milk, cheese, and condiments. Trans-fats (partially hydrogenated oils) can be found in margarine, snack foods, biscuits, baked goods, and more.

- Limit 2 grams of saturated fat per serving.
- Choose foods with 0 trans fat; avoid foods that list "partially hydrogenated oil" as part of the first five ingredients.
- Ultimate goal: <10-20 grams saturated and < than 1 gram trans-fat

SODIUM: Canned items and packet seasonings are notorious for adding unwanted salt to your daily eating plan. Too much sodium can lead to high blood pressure and fluid retention.

- Purchase low-sodium or no-salt-added canned goods
- Choose foods that contain 300 mg or less per serving (limit 200 mg if you have hypertension).
- Pre-packaged meals: <600 mg sodium
- Ultimate goal: <3,000 mg sodium per day (<2,000 if you have hypertension)

FIBER: Unfortunately most Americans don't get enough! The typical American diet contains less than 15 grams per day. Your ultimate goal is at least 25-35 grams. Best sources are fruits, veggies, cereal, and whole grains.

Strategies:

- Choose high-fiber alternatives such as 100-percent whole-grain breads or brown rice.
- Choose foods that contain 3 or more grams of fiber (aim for 5 grams when you buy cereal).
- Beans, peas, lentils, and corn have a type of fiber that helps lower cholesterol.

SUGAR: While no established guideline for sugar exists, most Americans consume too much. Milk, yogurt, and fruit have naturally occurring sugar. The Nutrition Facts label lumps both "natural" and "added sugars" together. Therefore, you may want to look at the ingredient list. If sugar is one of the first four ingredients, limit this food, especially if it has high-fructose corn syrup.

- 4 grams of sugar = 1 tsp of sugar. So if your favorite yogurt contains 40 grams of sugar for a 6-ounce container, that is equivalent to 10 teaspoons!

Use these strategies at least 85 percent of the time; you will be on your way to selecting healthier pre-packaged food. However, don't forget your "whole foods" always are the healthier option! Print out the information from the link below for more information!

http://www.cfsan.fda.gov/~dms/foodlab.html—for adults
http://www.kidshealth.org/kid/stay_healthy/food/labels.html—for children

Questions for the group

Ask members to discuss the following questions:

• Ask members to discuss the food labels they brought to class this week. Compare the labels.

• Discuss how planning ahead can be a valuable practice to keep you on the road to a healthy lifestyle.

• Discuss how to take this information and use it when you plan meals.

Individually this week

Ask members to thoughtfully and prayerfully consider these three questions. They may write their answers in the blanks provided.

• Rate yourself on the tips above (1=never 10=always). Derive an "action" plan as to how you can improve in at least one area this week.

• Evaluate your pantry using the guidelines from the food label. Are you surprised in what you find? Do you know of any pre-packaged foods that you now will avoid purchasing? If so, what would be a healthier replacement?

Class Lesson Week 6

Leader presentation

(The leader presents to the group the following lesson on evangelism.)

Both you and I walk on a spiritual journey. This spiritual journey began the day we became Christians—the day we believed and recognized Jesus as Savior (Rom. 10:9-13). Our journey will end at home—at our Father's house. Today we will begin our study of the spiritual discipline of evangelism. Ask the group members to turn to and read silently John 14:1-6.

For a little bit of context on this passage, this discussion between Jesus and His disciples occurs before his crucifixion. Jesus has met with his 12 disciples in the upper room; they have taken the last supper. As we studied in our week on service, He washes their feet and gives them a treasured teaching they will only fully understand and value after His death and resurrection.

When they first hear this message, it likely causes heartburn instead of joy, for their teacher tells them He will leave them. *What about the kingdom?* they likely wonder. *Aren't you the Messiah—the Christ?*

How disturbing. Your beloved teacher tells you He will leave you soon. What next? To say the least the disciples are confused and uncertain.

The disciples likely feel troubled or shaky. *What can we trust? On what can we rely?*

In John 14:1-4, Jesus gives a response. Ask group members to read these verses and answer these questions:

- **In John 14:1, Jesus gives two commands. What are they?**
- **Based on His word choice how certain are the statements Christ makes in John 14:2-3?**

Christ gives us 100-percent certainty that what He says is true.

Thomas asks a legitimate question based on uncertainty. "*Lord, we don't know where you are going, so how can we know the way?*" (John 14:5).

Jesus gives Thomas a direct answer, but He does not point to His teaching or tasks the disciples need to accomplish. He points to Himself. Jesus answers, "*I am the way and the truth and the life. No one comes to the Father except through me*" (John 14:6).

I find this verse most helpful when I share Christ with my friends. Most of them know about some of the teachings about Christ, but they are not always familiar with Scripture. They question whether Jesus really will reject others who choose alternative ways of salvation. John presents in his gospel a God of love who transforms the lives He encountered. A completely reliable message: believe and be saved. But John records Jesus' words in which He does not mince the truth. Jesus describes salvation in a way that is devoid of gray area. Salvation is found in Christ and Christ alone. Jesus clarifies how to find the only way of salvation—that is love. For another Scripture reference that supports this, ask class members to read Acts 4:12.

Jesus teaches repentance and salvation. He brings a new teaching, a new covenant, and because of His death and resurrection, He offers us a new life. But we cannot just accept Jesus' teachings as good. We must accept Jesus Christ as fully God and fully man—our only way of salvation.

Questions for the group

Ask members to discuss the following questions:

• If a friend or family member, asked whether you really thought Jesus was the only way, how would you respond?

• During the rest of class of the class time read portions of the Gospel of John together. Reading Scripture aloud promotes fellowship and discipleship within the church. Plan to separate the book into chapter segments and have everyone in the group read a segment. This gospel will highlight God's love and the salvation He offers. It also will provide clarity when you talk with friends or family about the salvation and new life Christ followers claim. Note: When I practice evangelism, I encourage people to read the Bible for themselves. I suggest they start with John.

(The leader then presents to the group the following health and fitness lesson.)

Have you ever had one of those "ah-ha!" moments that changed life forever? Five years ago I had such a moment. I was struggling and questioning God; I was asking "why" a series of painful events took place in my life. Anger and resentment—two emotions with which I was not accustomed to wrestling—kept me stuck in the past as I persistently asked "why?"

On a Florida beach, my "ah-ha" moment was revealed; it was simple but profound. The day was crowded and sunny; I was visiting a dear friend. Sitting on the beach I was unusually anxious, so I decided to walk up to the boardwalk and find a spot to pray. I broke down in tears; I was still wondering "why" I had to endure deep pain and feel so utterly lost. Suddenly time seemed to stand still; the Lord spoke directly to my heart. He seemed to say, "Julie, not *why?* but *WHAT NOW*?" I was so caught up in the "why?", I couldn't move forward to the "what now?" God had more to teach me and show me, but I was stuck in the past. That "ah-ha" moment was a turning point that led to healing, forgiveness, and a greater sense of purpose.

My hope for you is that you would continue to look forward and not back! If during the last six weeks you were not successful in making changes, this is OK; look forward to "WHAT NOW?"!

Questions for the group

Ask members to discuss the following questions. Members may write their personal answers in the spaces provided below.

What "barriers or obstacles" cause making a healthier lifestyle a priority to be difficult?

____

____

____

What strategies could I put into place to overcome these?

____

____

____

Individually this week

Ask members to thoughtfully and prayerfully consider this question. They may write their answers in the space provided.

• Identify what may motivate you to continue to focus on healthy eating and exercise habits.

____

____

____

____

Five P's for continued success

Ask members to follow along with you in their workbooks as you review the following concepts with them.

This is a review of the concepts discussed over the last six weeks. Try to apply one P at a time until you have achieved a healthier eating style at least 85-90 percent of the time. As a group take time to share ideas and offer encouragement!

1. Pre-Plan: This is the ultimate key to unlocking a life filled with healthier food choices. Pre-planning allows you to take control of what and where you choose to eat.

• Break(the) fast and eat often! This most-important meal will ensure your day is off to the right start by boosting your metabolism, providing mental acuity to conquer the day, and helping to stave off late-night munchies.

• **Be prepared for a snack attack!** Keep healthy snacks available to avoid the temptation.

2. Pre-Plate—and focus: Put everything on a plate before it touches your lips, so you mindfully acknowledge what you are eating. Chew your food well. This can help increase enjoyment of food, slow down the pace at which you eat, aid in digestion, and help you feel full more quickly.

• **Turn off the noise:** Take time to sit down at the table for meals. Consider listening to relaxing music.

• **Baggie it:** If the bag of chips or box of cookies is a danger zone, then get out the baggies and portion into individual servings!

• **Savor the flavor:** Test it out; practice this idea of mindful eating next time you eat. Experience flavors you never took time to appreciate before!

3. Portion Control: The concepts above can help with your portion control, but these guidelines will be effective in keeping portions reasonable.

• **Downsize:** Serve food on smaller plates. Use an 8- to 9-inch plate instead of the more typical 12-inch plate (restaurants often use a 15-inch plate!)

• **Pre-serve:** Instead of placing serving bowls on the table, serve food on individual plates. Don't go back for seconds, unless you want seconds on veggies!

• **Practice the 1/2, 1/4, 1/4 Rule!**

Select **lean protein** sources such as poultry, pork, beef, fish, and turkey, and limit it to only 1/4 of your plate (usually size of a deck of cards).

• **Whole grain carbohydrates** should fill the other 1/4 of your plate: Things such as brown rice, whole-wheat pasta, potatoes, corn, peas, beans, and legumes are excellent choices high in fiber and nutrients! Limit refined starched and sugars.

• 1/2 of your plate should be **full of color.** This is where your nutrient-packed vegetables fit in. This can include salads, steamed vegetables, vegetable salads made with low-fat dressings, or raw veggie sticks.

4. Pleasure: A variety of flavorful foods will help keep the meal fun and interesting and easy to achieve your wellness goals!

• **Have fun and make it easy!** Commit to trying a new fruit, vegetable, or grain weekly to jazz up your everyday fare. Be creative and involve the entire family.

5. Practice and Partner: Healthy habits take constant practice and partnership. Encouragement can be critical for success.

- Share your goals with someone who can help keep you "lovingly" accountable.
- Commit to learn more about nutrition, subscribe to a health journal, or read the "Healthy Living" section in the local paper to keep you focused on wellness
- Surround yourself with like-minded individuals who value health.

CELEBRATE—share your success!!!

May God bless as you strive to honor Him by keeping your body healthy and fit for service!

All of us involved in this project will pray that those who use this guide will achieve a healthy relationship with food and fitness for life while they discover a deeper and richer relationship with the Lord!

Appendix

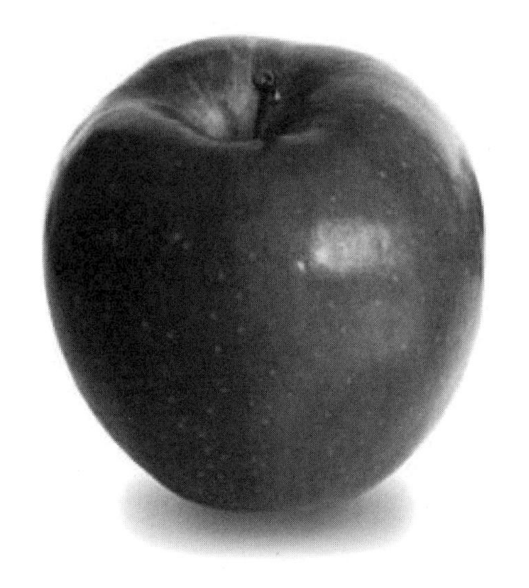

Activity Pyramid

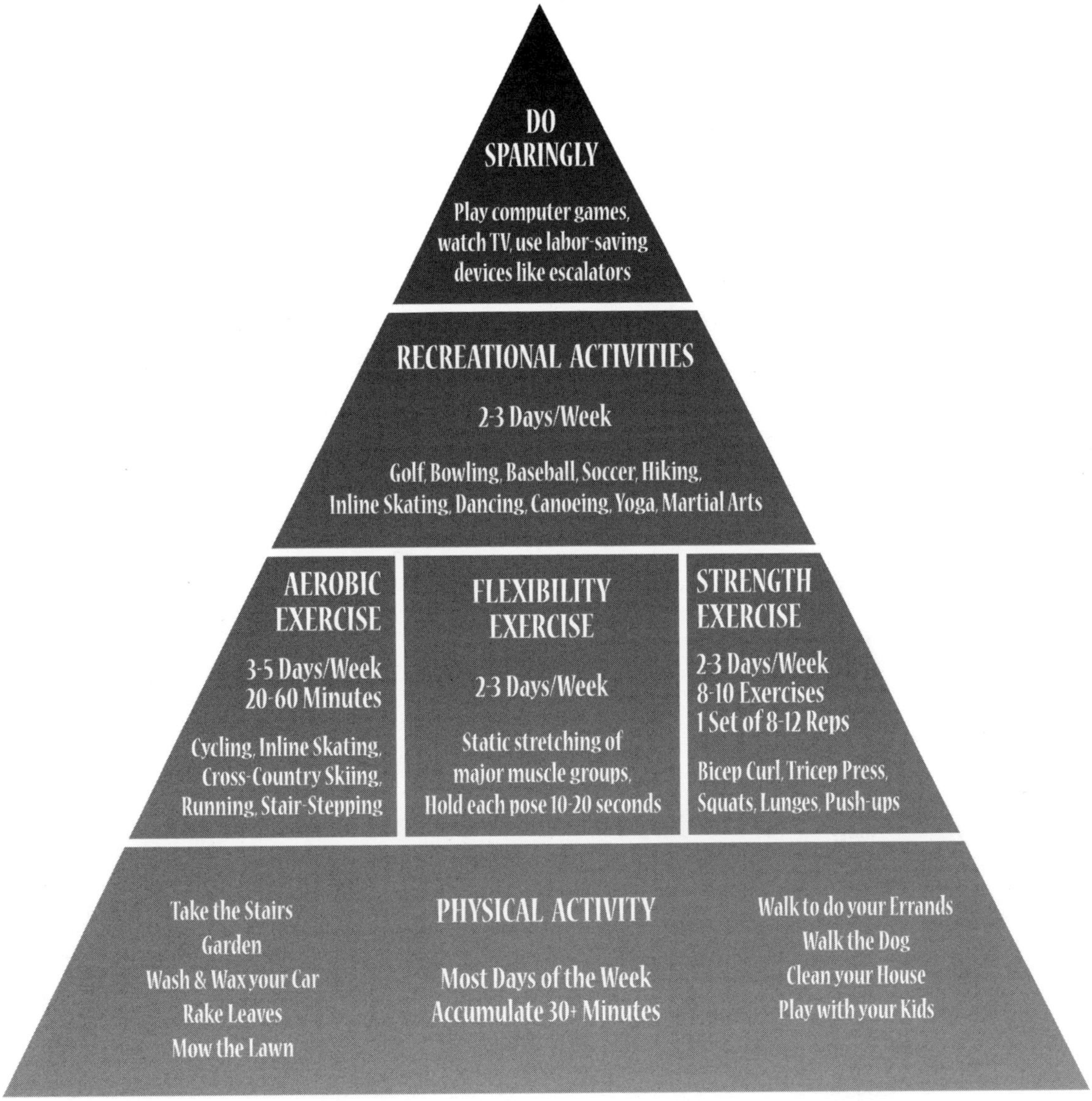

DO SPARINGLY

Play computer games, watch TV, use labor-saving devices like escalators

RECREATIONAL ACTIVITIES

2-3 Days/Week

Golf, Bowling, Baseball, Soccer, Hiking, Inline Skating, Dancing, Canoeing, Yoga, Martial Arts

AEROBIC EXERCISE

3-5 Days/Week
20-60 Minutes

Cycling, Inline Skating, Cross-Country Skiing, Running, Stair-Stepping

FLEXIBILITY EXERCISE

2-3 Days/Week

Static stretching of major muscle groups, Hold each pose 10-20 seconds

STRENGTH EXERCISE

2-3 Days/Week
8-10 Exercises
1 Set of 8-12 Reps

Bicep Curl, Tricep Press, Squats, Lunges, Push-ups

PHYSICAL ACTIVITY

Most Days of the Week
Accumulate 30+ Minutes

Take the Stairs
Garden
Wash & Wax your Car
Rake Leaves
Mow the Lawn

Walk to do your Errands
Walk the Dog
Clean your House
Play with your Kids

My Activity Pyramid

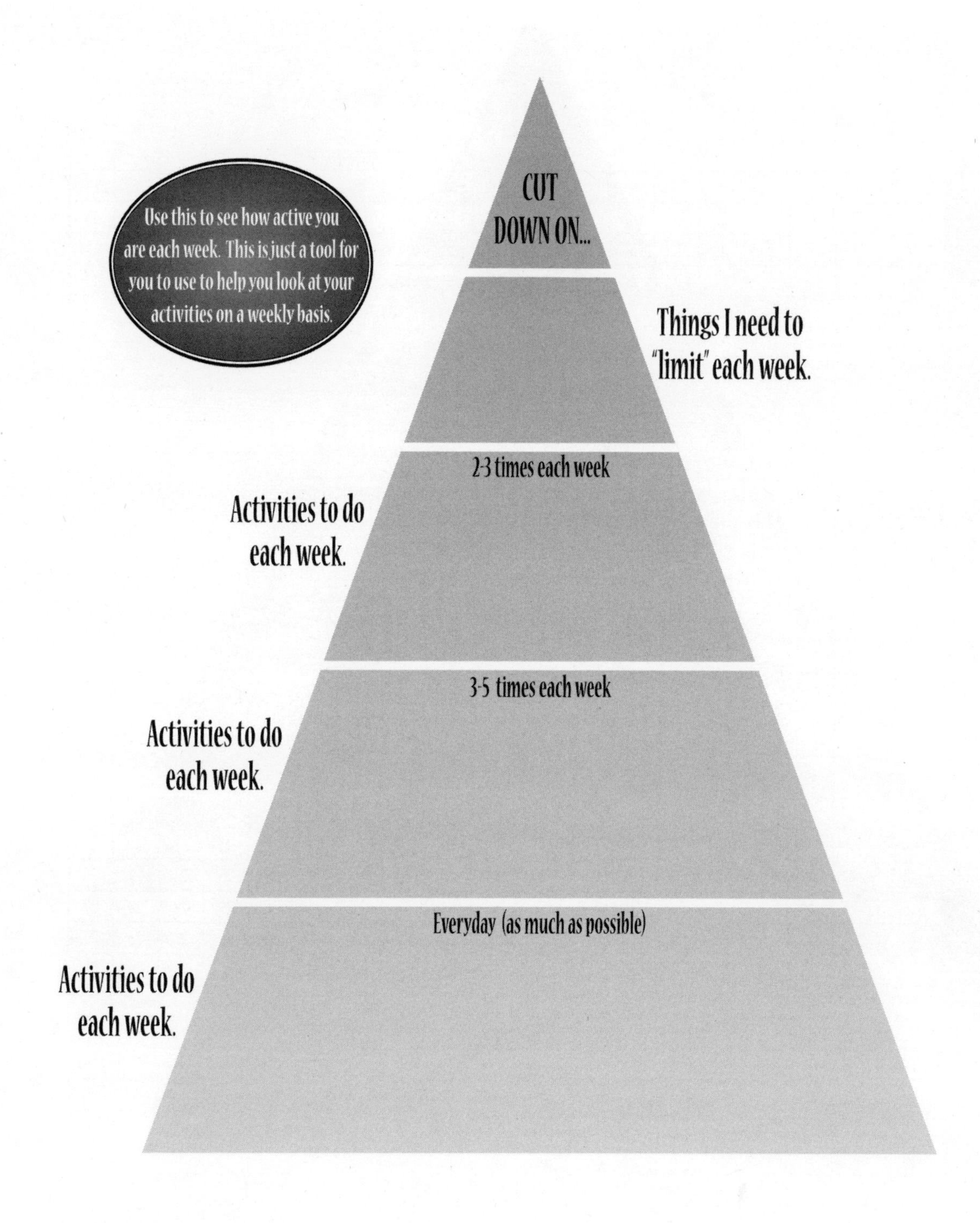

Body Mass Index Chart

Calculate Your Body Mass Index

BMI	Height (in)																		
	58	59	60	61	62	63	64	65	66	67	68	69	70	71	72	73	74	75	76
Weight (lbs)	4'10"	4'11"	5'0"	5'1"	5'2"	5'3"	5'4"	5'5"	5'6"	5'7"	5'8"	5'9"	5'10"	5'11"	6'0"	6'1"	6'2"	6'3"	6'4"
100	21	20	20	19	18	18	17	17	16	16	15	15	14	14	14	13	13	13	12
105	22	21	21	20	19	19	18	18	17	16	16	16	15	15	14	14	14	13	13
110	23	22	22	21	20	20	19	18	18	17	17	16	16	15	15	15	14	14	13
115	24	23	23	22	21	20	20	19	19	18	18	17	17	16	16	15	15	14	14
120	25	24	23	23	22	21	21	10	19	19	18	18	17	17	16	16	15	15	15
125	26	25	24	24	23	22	22	21	20	18	18	17	17	16	16	15	15	15	15
130	27	26	25	25	24	23	22	22	21	20	20	19	19	18	18	17	17	16	16
135	28	27	26	26	25	24	23	23	22	21	21	20	19	19	18	18	17	17	16
140	29	28	27	27	26	25	24	23	23	22	21	21	20	20	19	19	18	18	17
145	30	29	28	27	27	26	25	24	23	23	22	21	21	20	20	19	19	18	18
150	31	30	29	28	27	27	26	25	24	24	23	22	22	21	20	20	19	19	18
155	32	31	30	29	28	28	27	26	25	24	24	23	22	22	21	20	20	19	19
160	34	32	31	30	29	28	28	27	26	25	24	24	23	22	22	21	21	20	20
165	35	33	32	31	30	29	28	28	27	26	25	24	24	23	22	22	21	21	20
170	36	34	33	32	31	30	29	28	27	27	26	25	24	24	23	22	22	21	21
175	37	35	34	33	32	31	30	29	28	27	27	26	25	24	24	23	23	22	21
180	38	36	35	34	33	32	31	30	29	28	27	27	26	25	24	24	23	23	22
185	39	37	36	35	34	33	32	31	30	29	28	27	27	26	25	24	24	23	23
190	40	38	37	36	35	34	33	32	31	30	29	28	27	27	26	25	24	24	23
195	41	39	38	37	36	35	34	33	32	31	30	29	28	27	27	26	25	24	24
200	42	40	39	38	37	36	34	33	32	31	30	30	29	28	27	26	26	25	24
205	43	41	40	39	38	36	35	34	33	32	31	30	29	29	28	27	26	26	25
210	44	43	41	40	38	37	36	35	34	33	32	31	30	29	29	28	27	26	26
215	45	44	42	41	39	38	37	36	35	34	33	32	31	30	29	28	28	27	26
220	46	45	43	42	40	39	38	37	36	35	34	33	32	31	30	29	28	28	27
225	47	46	44	43	41	40	39	38	36	35	34	33	32	31	31	30	29	28	27
230	48	47	45	44	42	41	40	38	37	36	35	34	33	32	31	30	30	29	28
235	49	48	46	44	43	42	40	39	38	37	36	35	34	33	32	31	30	29	29
240	50	49	47	45	44	43	41	40	39	38	37	36	35	34	33	32	31	30	29
245	51	50	48	46	45	43	42	41	40	38	37	36	35	34	33	32	32	31	30
250	52	51	49	47	46	44	43	42	40	39	38	37	36	35	34	33	32	31	30
255	53	52	50	48	47	45	44	43	41	40	39	38	37	36	35	34	33	32	31
260	54	53	51	49	48	46	45	43	42	41	40	38	37	36	35	34	33	33	32
265	56	54	52	50	49	47	46	44	43	42	40	39	38	37	36	35	34	33	32
270	57	55	53	51	49	48	46	45	44	42	41	40	39	38	37	36	35	34	33

Hip-to-Waist Ratio

1. Step One. Stand with your stomach relaxed.
2. Step Two. Find the narrowest point at your waist and measure. Write down the measurement.
3. Step Three. Find the widest point of your hips and buttocks and measure. Write down this measurement.
4. Step Four. Divide the calculation from step 2 by the calculation from step 3. This is your waist-to-hip ratio.

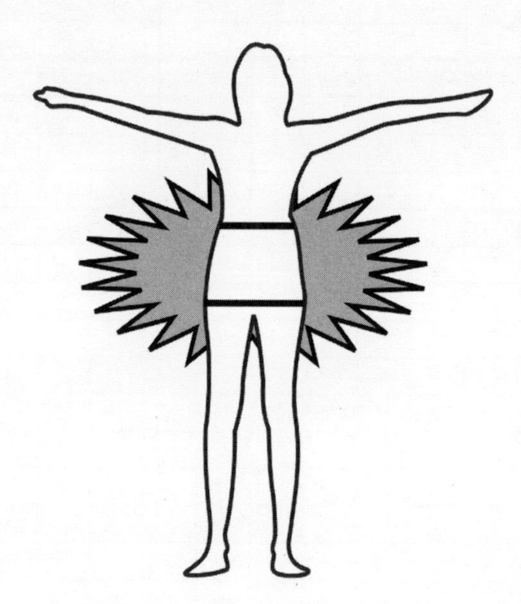

	acceptable		unacceptable		
	excellent	**good**	**average**	**high**	**extreme**
male	**<0.85**	**0.85 - 0.90**	**0.90 - 0.95**	**0.95 - 1.00**	**> 1.00**
female	**<0.75**	**0.75 - 0.80**	**0.80 - 0.85**	**0.85 - 0.90**	**> 0.90**

Target Heart Rate

You can use the following formula to estimate your exercise heart rate,

Constant:	220	
Your age:		
Subtract age from constant; this equals estimated maximum heart rate:		
Your resting heart rate (count pulse for 1 minute):		
Subtract resting heart rate from estimated maximum heart rate:		
Multiply by:	60%	80%
Equals:		
Add resting heart rate:		
Equals exercise heart rate:		
	Target Zone	

SMART Goals

How to set **SMART** goals

Specific
Measurable
Action-based
Realistic
Time-line

Being ***specific*** about the actions or behavior you would like to take to reach your vision is important. This will increase your level of success. Be specific about the details of ***when*** and ***how*** you will accomplish your goal.

Set a ***time frame*** in which to accomplish your goal. This may help avoid putting it off.

Goals need to be ***measurable*** so that success can be determined.

Break down goals into ***behaviors or actions*** that will help move you closer to your ultimate goal.

Ensure that goals you set for yourself are ***realistic!*** Realistic goal-setting is essential for success because if success follows . . . then you will be more likely to move forward to reach your ultimate goal! Success builds self-confidence and self-efficacy. Nothing inhibits the change process more than does setting ***un***realistic goals.

A **SMART** goal is one that you feel you are fully in charge of accomplishing through specific steps!

Examples:

"I will eat a healthy breakfast on Monday, Wednesday, and Friday at 8 a.m."

"I will get at least seven hours of sleep on Saturday, Sunday, and Wednesday nights by going to bed at 10 p.m."

"I will substitute 2 tablespoons of light salad dressing for regular ranch dressing on my salad this week."

"I will include a cup of vegetables at dinner five times this week."

SNACKS THAT WILL *FUEL* AND *FILL* YOU FOR SUCCESS!

• celery sticks, apple, or banana topped with all-natural peanut butter (1-2 tablespoons)

• low-fat cheese cubes with six triscuits or 10-12 pita chips dipped in light cheese

• 1/4 cup tuna salad or chicken salad with five-six crackers

• fruit yogurt cup—add in fresh fruit or nuts for a boost

• 1/4 cup almond, walnuts, or peanuts and handful of pretzels (toss in a baggie for an on-the-go snack

• vegetable sticks (carrot, cucumber, pepper, celery) dipped in low-fat ranch dressing and 15 blue corn chips

• 1/2 cup fruit with 1/2 cup light cottage cheese

• half of a turkey/tuna/ham sandwich on whole-wheat bread with a slice of avocado

• yogurt and granola (1 cup yogurt, 1/4 cup granola)

• chicken, turkey, or ham slices wrapped in a mini whole-wheat tortilla—add 1 tablespoon guacamole for a burst of flavor

• fiber-rich cereal mixed with nuts (3/4 cup cereal, 1/4 cup nuts)

•1/2 peanut butter and jelly sandwich)

• 17 soy crisps (a favorite is barbecue flavor) with 1/4 cup almonds (or your choice nuts)

• whole fruit with one to two ounces of cheese; kiwi, mango, papaya, prickly pear, plum—try something new

• whole-wheat crackers or tomato basil wheat thins (four to six) with string cheese and carrot sticks

• granola bar (suggest looking for one with 7-14 grams of protein, a minimum of 3 grams of fiber, 0 trans fat).

• fruit smoothie in an insulated bottle (blend up at home and take on the go)

• tortilla filled with hummus (three tablespoons) and your choice of veggies

STAGES OF CHANGES

The Stages of Readiness to Change is a vehicle that can help assess where you are in the journey toward changing lifestyle habits. It may help you gain understanding of the process of change and may assist with achieving *lasting change*. Moving through the various changes is typical. Attempt to identify what stage best describes you when initiating healthy eating and exercise habits is concerned.

Stage 1: Pre-contemplation—"I won't/I can't"
You may believe that nothing is wrong with the behavior in question. You have no desire to change.

Stage 2: Contemplation—" I might"
You are thinking about changing behavior but are not ready to commit. You may consider how life would be altered if you were to make changes; perhaps you are weighing the pros and cons.

Stage 3: Preparation—"I will"
You are ready to make that first step to change the behavior and plan to do so in the near future. Decision-making and ongoing commitment to the decision to change continues throughout this stage. While in this stage, make plans that will work for you and that will help you to maintain your commitment.

Stage 4: Action—"I am"
You are actively engaged in changing the behavior and are implementing a plan. Experiencing conflicting feelings about the change is normal. You may miss your old lifestyle. This stage requires the greatest amount of action and commitment of time and energy. Reaffirm your decision by believing in your own ability to influence your achievement.

Stage 5: Maintenance—"I still am"
You no longer need to actively work on changing behavior. You are concentrating on the gains made during the action stage and are striving to prevent relapse. Lapses or temporary setbacks are common! Here is where concentrating on your "motivators" can help you from relapsing.

Stage 6: Relapse—"I am going to get back on track"
You may temporarily go back to old behaviors. Once a relapse has occurred, you may need to go back to an earlier stage and begin processing through the stages of change again. A relapse should be considered a setback, not a failure. A relapse presents an opportunity to practice at slipping up and proving you can get back on track!

BIBLIOGRAPHY FOR APPENDIX

Fahey, Thomas D., Paul M. Insel, Walton T. Roth. *Fit and Well.* (Mountain View, CA:Mayfield Publishing Company, 1999).

Kravitz, Len. *Anybody's Guide to Total Fitness.* (Dubuque, IA: Kendall/Hunt Publishing Company, 1995)

Corbin, Charles B., Gregory J. Welk, William R. Corbin, Karen A. Welk. *Concepts of Fitness and Wellness.* (New York: McGrawHill, 2008).

Robbins, Gwen, Debbie Powers, Sharon Burgess. *A Wellness Way of Life* (New York: McGraw Hill, 2008).

Rippe, James. *One-Mile Walking Test.* Walk100-Walking Test and Speed Calculator website.

COLLABORATORS

Don and Carol Mathus

Don and Carol Mathus recently retired from 30-plus years of teaching physical education. They are developing a wellness program for the staff at their church, Lake Pointe, in Rockwall, TX.

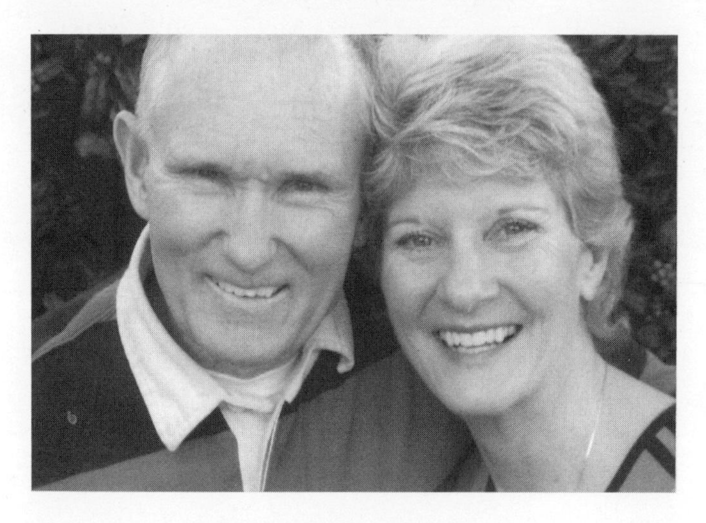

Julie Bender

Julie Bender is a registered dietitian and certified wellness coach who resides in Dallas and has been in practice for more than 10 years (*jbender7@tx.rr.com*). She helps others achieve personal health and nutrition goals through education, motivational counseling, and public speaking.

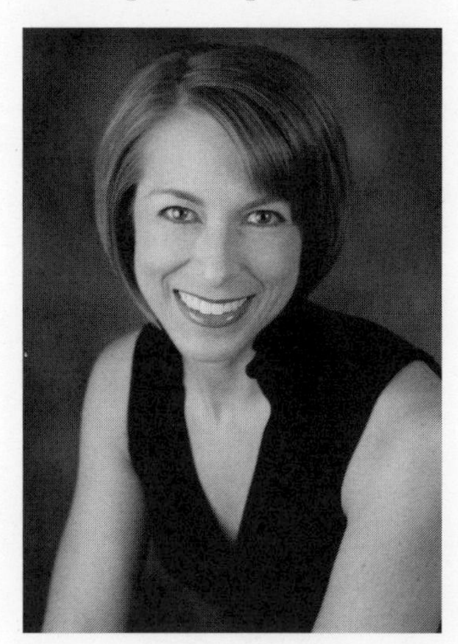